An Unconventional Death

A Novel

By Dorothy Mai

This book is a work of fiction. Although The Texas Institute for Rehabilitation and Research (TIRR) and the University of Houston, College of Optometry (UHCO) are actual organizations, their use in this story is purely fictional. Names, characters, businesses, organizations, and incidents are a product of the author's imagination or are used fictitiously. Any resemblance to actual events or persons, living or dead, is entirely coincidental.

For Howard and Sera who believe in me
and for hardworking optometrists everywhere.

Tea tree *noun* : 2 any of various melaleucas (especially *Melaleuca alternifolia*) with aromatic leaves that yield an essential oil used especially as an antiseptic

--Merriam Webster Dictionary

Chapter 1

The sound of the clock ticking was deafening in the quiet of the 8 by 12 square ft room. Perhaps it was the echoes reverberating off the stark, white walls and metallic casings of the exam room equipment that made it appear so loud. It had already been a full five minutes since I had asked the patient to read the line of letters on the screen a mere 10 ft across the room. At this point, I was afraid the young man had fallen asleep.

It had happened before. Only that patient was a 75-year-old gentleman who had unwisely scheduled his exam on a warm afternoon and close to his regular nap time. Apparently, the room lights were dimmed too low during the exam and the coziness of the small space contributed to the sleepy atmosphere. Evidently, I had also been speaking too quietly. That 75-year-old patient informed me that my voice had put him to sleep because it was soft and lilting like a lullaby. I had taken it as a learning experience and a compliment of sorts since my husband, Fred, told me that my singing sounded more like Indian Bollywood music than the enchanting country ballads of Ms. Shania Twain.

Therefore, likening my voice to a soothing lullaby was a step up.

I have since kept the room at a modest illumination level and forced myself to speak louder and with more authority. Serendipitously, these changes have also encouraged my patients to have more confidence in me, which in turn has boosted my own confidence when dealing with the public. Don't get me wrong, I love the science and art of optometry. Making observations, collecting data, putting it all together to find the right diagnosis to solve people's eye problems; it's all part of why I became an optometrist. The years of education and training I received in school, on clinical rotations, from mentors and in the trenches at work have made me a good eye doctor. My position allows me to help people and helping people brings me fulfillment. However, I detest confrontation. When choosing to enter the field, I didn't have a clue as to how much of it I would have to deal with as a health care provider. But then again, maybe it's gotten worse over the years.

My guess for this change in attitudes and treatment of healthcare providers is likely to do with a change in the speed of living life. In this modern age, information can be acquired at the speed of typing into a computer. Material things can be bought and sold without having to speak to a living being. Medical science is so advanced that drugs and surgery have gone beyond simply treating illness and pain. Every day brings new ways to enhance our appearances or to try and cheat aging and death with a simple snip, prick, swallow, or application. And so, when proper care and treatment take a little more time than may be convenient, tempers flare and I retreat behind the mask of quiet insecurity.

The other aspect of optometry for which I was not fully prepared, or particularly enjoy, is dealing with the American healthcare system. Don't get me started on co-pays. In private practice it's not enough to provide healthcare. We are small businesses. We must navigate insurance mazes, worry about competition, rent, staffing, and paying our inventory and lab bills on time to keep the lights on. It is the price of being independent, but these are the constant worries that live in my subconscious and travel with me on my daily commute to work.

These thoughts have led to periods of melancholy. In my years of practice, I have found that patients who choose to be unkind to their healthcare providers do not fully comprehend or appreciate what they do. I understand that sometimes people are just having a bad day, but in my current state of mind, it can be too much. I hoped that today was not going to be one of those days.

This patient had already shown up ten minutes late and now the eye exam was taking longer than it should for a seemingly healthy, young man. As much as I wanted to give him all the time he needed, I had to be mindful of keeping on schedule. The staff had let me know that my next patient was already here, had finished filling out paperwork and asked how long the exam would take while she was checking the time on her watch. I wasn't even halfway through this exam. Second patient of the day and I was already feeling stressed.

This patient was 17 years old. He appeared athletic and in the prime of life. His past medical history showed no indication of physical or mental illness. He seemed fine five minutes ago, and yet something was surely going on in that teenage mind of his. I finally had to break the silence and ask again for the third time.

"Ahem, so can you read the letters for me?" I prodded. Then I rephrased, "Can you *see* the letters? Or anything at all?"

He finally cleared his throat and spoke. "What are we doing again? You want me to read letters?"

"Tell you what, let's take a little break," I suggested as I pulled the phoropter away from his face. "Is there something on your mind that might be distracting you?" I inquired gently while observing his demeanor more closely.

"What do you mean?" he replied confused.

"Is everything all right at home? Anyone sick?" I probed.

"No, everyone is doing okay at home," he responded. His eyes roamed around the room as if he was considering whether to share more.

"How about school? You're a senior this year, right?"

"Yes, I am," he replied simply and with less enthusiasm than one would expect.

"Are you nervous about it?"

"Well, I guess maybe a little."

Aha, maybe something there.

"Do you want to talk about it?" I asked. I was aware of the time ticking by, but I had to get to the bottom of this peculiar behavior.

"I guess I *have* been feeling some pressure lately. I play football and I really want to play college ball at one of the big twelve schools. So, I've been putting in extra practice time and staying in the game maybe longer than I should. I mean I want to do well for recruiters, but in the last few games I found myself not feeling right afterwards. I'm the quarterback so everyone wants to take me down. Since it's recruitment season, all the guys are playing extra hard, and I have gotten sacked a lot lately. I had some trouble getting up after the last takedown and I felt out of it. I don't even remember what happened in the last quarter of the game."

"I see," I replied concerned with this new bit of information. "Was your vision blurry? Were you seeing double or light sensitive?"

He thought for a moment. "Come to think of it, the lights did seem really bright."

"Painfully bright, like you couldn't look at them?" I continued.

"Yes, I had trouble opening my eyes and when I did, it was blurry and when I looked at my hands, maybe it did seem like there were more of them than there should be. I also felt off balance, like I couldn't walk straight."

"Blurred and distorted vision can affect your balance. Sounds like you may even have had a concussion," I surmised. "How long did you feel that way?"

"All night after the game. It was better the next day after some sleep."

"Did you tell your parents about this?"

"They knew I got hit hard, so they just told me to take it easy that night. I didn't really tell them about the specific problems. I didn't want my mom to worry."

"It's understandable that you want to push yourself to achieve your goals, but you shouldn't sacrifice your physical or mental health. How do you think your parents would feel if you took some time off from football to fully recover?"

"I don't know if I can do that right now. The university recruiters will be coming in a week or so. They want me to do well and get scholarships. My dad got one to Texas A & M and wants me to do the same."

"Have you told him about how you've been feeling after the games?"

"I mean I tried, but he would say I just got my bell rung and I should shake it off."

"What about your mom?"

"She noticed that I didn't seem to see things well and I was having trouble concentrating on my schoolwork. That's why she wanted me to get my eyes checked."

I nodded approvingly.

"Yes, that was very good of her to have you get checked out. Tell you what, let's go take detailed photos of the back of your eyes, so we can better assess if there is any damage."

"Okay doc. Whatever you say," the young man said with a smile. "I appreciate you taking the time."

After my assistant took OCT and retinal photos, I pulled them up to examine them while my patient sat looking a bit dazed by the bright lights of the equipment. He seemed to be having a harder time recovering from it than one would expect for a young and healthy individual. Upon examination, some areas of the retina showed changes consistent with trauma. Thank goodness the macula, the central area of the retina responsible for detailed vision, was intact. Although there were no indications of a break or tear anywhere, there were small hemorrhages in the periphery.

"We should put drops in your eyes to dilate them," I stated.

"Actually, I have football practice after this, so I'd rather not."

I was just about to protest when a knock on the exam room door stopped me. I went to see who it was. It was Diya, my assistant, with a harried look on her face.

"Um, the patient's mother wants to know how much longer it will be. Her son needs to go to football practice soon. Also, the next patient is getting upset. She wants to know if it will be soon or else, she's going to leave."

"Right," I exhaled anxiously. "Please tell them each about ten more minutes. Thanks."

Moving quickly, I was able to finish the rest of the eye exam in that time. All other aspects of his eyes were within normal limits. The power of youth was on my side. Now the harder part, a conversation with mom. I went to the optical where the patient's mother was waiting and asked her to come into the exam room. She followed me back into the room.

"So does he need glasses?" she asked directly.

"Well, the good news is he doesn't have a significant refractive error."

"What does that mean?"

"If you have a refractive error, that means the optical structures of the eyes don't focus light correctly causing you to either be near-sighted, far-sighted or have astigmatism and need glasses to correct it."

"So, you're saying he does need glasses?"

"I'm saying he doesn't need glasses to correct his vision, that part is fine. However, in our discussions he mentioned receiving some head trauma during his football activities which has caused some symptoms of visual disturbance."

"What kind of disturbance?"

"Some light sensitivity, which some tinted lenses will help with if he continues to have this problem."

"Don't most people have light sensitivity in the sun?"

"True, but he reports pain to light, especially after getting knocked in the head. He also has transient double and distorted vision. I'm not a neurologist but it seems that he also has some cognitive confusion after the head trauma."

"You didn't tell me this Mike," she confronted her son.

"I didn't want you to worry. Dad said it was just because I got my bell rung. It was better the next day."

"Your father didn't tell me this either. What else have you two been keeping from me?"

"It's nothing mom," he insisted perhaps regretting saying anything.

"Actually, it is something. It sounds very much like he may have had a concussion, which is a mild traumatic brain injury. I have taken some detailed photos of the back of his eye to make sure there aren't any physical damages or changes. Blood spots consistent with trauma can be seen."

"Brain injury?" she exclaimed, shocked. "Are you telling me he could have brain injury from playing football?"

"I would recommend he go to a neurologist to confirm that he had a concussion and receive treatment if needed. Certainly, you can understand that with repeated hits to the head, the brain will be affected. How much, I can't say because that is not my area of expertise. However, if he has had a concussion, it would be best for Mike to rest to fully recover."

"So, are you saying that he definitely had a concussion?" she asked, visibly getting upset.

"Well, no not exactly. I can only say it is a possibility. Again, I'm not a neurologist but based on the trauma to his eyes, it would be best to investigate further to confirm or rule it out and treat it accordingly."

"So, if you're saying you can't diagnose if someone has had a concussion or not, why are you even telling me about it?"

"Well ma'am, I'm just trying to alert you to all the signs and potential issues so that you can make a decision that would be best for Mike's health."

I swallowed hard, feeling like I was digging myself into a giant hole. When will I learn to stay in my lane? Why didn't I just stick to the glasses?

"If you are interested in the current research and connections between football, concussions and brain injury, I could gather them up and forward them to you as well as other resources."

I could see by her expressions and body language that she was growing impatient.

"So, what I'm hearing is that you really have no experience with someone who has brain trauma?"

"Ma'am, I'm not a neurologist, so I'm not qualified to diagnose or treat brain trauma. However, I did do a clinical rotation at the Texas Institute for Rehabilitation and Research (TIRR) during my Low Vision residency. During that time, I did perform eye and vision assessments on patients who had traumatic brain injury."

"Well then give me a straight answer. Does he have any problems with his eyes or not?"

"Yes, of course. I apologize for the confusion. He does not need prescription glasses, but he does have some other visual symptoms, such as the light sensitivity for which sunglasses will help. There's no treatment for his mild retinal bleeding now. With time and rest they should resolve. We will monitor him closely. I recommend he return for a follow up in a day or two. Come back right away if there are more or worsening symptoms."

I should have really stopped there, but if I can help someone, I felt compelled to try.

"It's just, I'm sure Mike is a talented football player, but perhaps you might consider if continuing to play it at this time is the best thing for him," I said as neutrally as I could. I was trying to tread lightly. This was Texas after all. Football is a way of life.

"Uh huh. Well, thank you for your opinion, but I think we will make that decision ourselves. Let's go son," she commanded clearly agitated as she hustled her son from the room.

"Mrs. Stableson, I didn't mean to upset you. I just wanted you to know enough to make informed decisions. We both want the best for Mike."

"What's best for Mike right now is playing football. I just needed you to tell me if he needed glasses or not."

"I understand ma'am. But the eyes don't work on their own. You must take care of the whole person as well."

"So now you're a therapist too? What are you going to offer me next? Acupuncture? Incense and chanting?"

She motioned for him to follow her out of the exam door. Those last comments stung a little. Were there racial undertones? Nevertheless, I could see I wasn't getting anywhere with mom. Perhaps a different tactic.

"Mike, does the coach do any screenings for concussions during play time?" I asked following after them.

"I don't think so," he replied hesitantly. "He asks if I'm okay and then tells me to shake it off."

"Perhaps Mrs. Stableson you could speak to the coach to add concussion screenings during play time to make sure Mike gets pulled from the game if it happens," I suggested hurriedly trying to squeeze in more counseling while I still had them in the office. Mrs. Stableson was scrambling to get her credit card out to pay at this point.

"I don't tell the coach how to do his job," she snapped. "But I will say, you should stick to yours."

"What do you mean?" I asked, surprised by the accusation.

"I mean maybe you should stick to just looking at eyes instead of trying to play brain surgeon."

And with that, she snatched the receipt from Dora, my receptionist. She grabbed Mike by the arm and left in a huff.

"Wow. That spun out of control fast," I declared feeling deflated.

"Well, you did what you could. Some people don't want to hear what's good for them. Dr. Trí the next patient is in room two. New patient, and she's not in a good mood either," Adriana, my manager, informed me with little sympathy.

She was trying to keep me on schedule. She heard the commotion and came out to help.

"Right. Keep it moving," I complied looking at my watch and trying to prepare for the next verbal onslaught that was bound to come. I was fifteen minutes behind. Inconvenient yes, but not *that* bad. How upset could she be?

I knocked on the exam door before opening it as is my custom to make sure I don't walk in on someone in a compromising position.

"Hello Ms. Moody. How are you today?" I asked pleasantly while walking into the exam room.

"I was better before I came in here," she hissed. "And younger too. I have been waiting a really, long time. You're lucky I didn't just leave."

"Yes, I'm so sorry about the delay. It couldn't be helped," I apologized trying to diffuse the situation. For such a small office as mine, bedside manner was my big selling point.

"Do you even know what you're doing?" she asked as she looked me up and down. "You don't look old enough to be a doctor. How long have you been doing this doctor... Try is it? Thigh Try?"

"It's doctor Thi Trí ma'am. Pronounced "tea tree", you know like the essential oil that has many natural health benefits. And I assure you that I may look young, but I've been doing this for almost ten years."

It was eight years, but I think rounding up was justified to reassure this patient. It probably didn't help that my hair currently had streaks of lavender highlights in it. An unfortunate mishap from my hairdresser that I hadn't had time to correct. I tried to hide it by tying my hair back in a ponytail. A sleek hair bun would have been more professional looking, but I had neither the time nor talent for such an endeavor.

"Hmm," she hummed not looking wholly convinced. "Well, I guess since you're here we might as well go ahead."

"Wonderful," I proclaimed, forcing a smile. "How are your eyes doing?"

"Well, they could be better. Lately I haven't been able to read anything clearly. It's all blurry up close and I don't know why. Two years ago, my vision was perfectly fine."

I quickly looked through the medical and ocular history that she filled out which was all normal. Then I glanced at her age. Forty-five. This was not going to be a fun discussion.

"Could you tell me if you have been using any optical aids such as eyeglasses for either distance or near and particularly for reading?"

"I don't use any glasses. My eyes are perfect. I just use a magnifier when I need to read something. But that's why I'm here. I need you to tell me what's wrong with my vision and to fix it."

"I see," I replied politely. "Let's start with checking your vision."

I handed her a cover paddle which looks like a large, flattened spoon.

"Could you please cover your left eye?"

She covered her right eye.

"Okay, well how about you look to the end of the room at the screen straight ahead and read for me the smallest line of letters you can see."

She proceeded to read the largest letter and then the next line down and stopped.

"Is that the smallest you can see, or can you see some letters in the next line below?"

"Well, yes, I can see all the way down to the smallest. Well almost the smallest. That line is too small. Who can see that small?"

"You're able to read the 20/25 line, that's not too bad."

"But isn't 20/20 the best? I'm going blind."

"No ma'am, I've worked with visually impaired and blind individuals. You are definitely not going blind."

The rest of the exam went on in this manner. At the end of the exam, I determined that she was hyperopic, or far-sighted, with presbyopia. The eye health exam was unremarkable.

"Ms. Moody your eyes are healthy however you do have a prescription for eyeglasses."

"Glasses? Why do I need glasses if my eyes are healthy?"

"When I say the eyes are healthy, I mean they are free of disease. However, the eyes are not just blood and tissue, they have optical components too. Think of the eye as a camera. To get a clear picture, the lenses in front need the correct power to focus correctly. This is the case for your eyes."

"Is that why I can hardly see anything up close?"

"Yes. You are now presbyopic, which is what happens to the eyes as we get older than forty. The condition is called presbyopia, a term originating from Greek meaning "old eyes"."

"Now you're calling me old!" she cried indignantly.

"No ma'am, I'm not calling you old, just your eyes. I mean, you are over forty, so your eyes have changed. It's normal. Our natural lens ages with us and doesn't work as well anymore. Therefore, we have to rely on optical aids such as reading glasses or multifocal glasses for up close."

"I don't like glasses," she replied with a frown.

"Glasses are the easiest way to treat presbyopia and are very effective. "

"Well," she conceded. "That sounds like what the last doctor told me."

"Oh, what did the last doctor tell you?"

"He said I was getting old and needed to wear reading glasses or bifocals, but not like the way you did. I didn't believe him and thought he was insulting and just trying to sell me glasses, so I didn't get any. Is there a surgery I could get to fix my eyes?"

"No."

She frowned.

"But I don't want to wear glasses," she insisted.

"If you don't mind my asking, what is it about glasses that bothers you? You may think I'm biased, but I think they're one of the most ingenious inventions of humankind. Simple, effective, portable, accessible."

"If you must know, I just don't like the way they look on me. They make me feel old and are heavy on my nose."

"Hmm," I responded unconsciously noticing the large pair of sunglasses resting on her purse in the chair near the door. "Let me show you something."

14

I reached into my desk drawer and pulled out a trial frame that we use to test spectacle prescriptions. I popped in the lenses for her reading prescription and put them on her face. I handed her a reading card and asked her to read it. She obliged and read everything perfectly.

"What do you think?" I asked.

"The vision is good. I haven't seen that well up close in years. It still feels a little heavy on my nose."

"Yes, these frames are too heavy. However, if you will follow me to the optical, our optician John will help you find a pair of glasses that will not only be much lighter on your nose but will look fashionable and fabulous."

"Okay, I like red. I wear a lot of red," she replied as she got out of the chair, picked up her purse and followed me out of the exam room.

I smiled to myself and was glad that I could at least solve Ms. Moody's problem. Small victories. I looked for John and guided Ms. Moody to him.

"John, Ms. Moody is needing some chic glasses to compliment her face. It's her first pair of prescription glasses. Please take good care of her," I instructed him while handing him her chart.

"Of course," he said cheerfully. "Ms. Moody, I think we need something to accentuate those beautiful brown eyes of yours."

John was a great salesman and optician. I was lucky to have him after a string of other opticians, good and bad, had left for higher paying positions at chain stores or bigger practices after training with us. Good employee retention is difficult in the struggle against chains and private equity firms.

Business had been on and off lately. Our shopping center lost its grocery store. It was our anchor business for foot traffic. We were down to the Mexican taqueria to our right, the Chinese restaurant to our left and the small, free-standing coffee shop in the parking lot in front of us.

I tried not to think about the business side of the office as it always brought me down. It almost led me to divorce. Trying to repay the bank loan for the office build out along with my student loans led to many sleepless nights and frayed nerves. Words were said that could not be unsaid. Although things got better as patients came, we stayed together by agreeing to not talk about the office at home. I went to the reception desk to see about my next patient.

"Is the next patient ready?" I asked Dora.

"Bad news doc. The family of four cancelled. Apparently, their insurance was just a discount plan, so they decided to go to a discount chain in the mall."

"That is bad news," I replied.

That cancellation wiped out the rest of my morning appointments. Looks like another break-even month.

The bell dinged on the front office door. I looked up to see who had come in. It was a uniformed policeman. What now?

Chapter 2

I led the police officer to an exam room for a private conversation.

"Hi doc. How's business?" he asked sitting down in the exam chair.

"Oh, you know, another day, another forty cents on the dollar from insurance reimbursements. What can I do for you Officer Custos?" I replied cordially.

"So formal today. I'm practically your brother-in-law," he replied.

"That would be true Jaime, if Lan were my biological sister instead of my best friend."

"I've seen you two together, you're pretty much sisters."

This was true. Although I had a brother, I had always wanted a sister. So ever since I helped exonerate her from false accusations of stealing a classmate's pencil box in first grade, Lan Nguyen and I have been as close as sisters. She was also my hairdresser, which was why I agreed to let her try out the grey hair coloring on me that younger clients were requesting. I have no idea why young people would want to color their hair to make it look older. In my case, the daily questions about my age were enough to let Lan practice on me. I didn't think a paying customer would have liked this streaky lavender look, but then again what do I know about being edgy.

Jaime looked at my hair with an amused smile and pointed at it.

"Lan's handy work?" he asked.

"Yep."

"Not sure it's the right shade for an eye doctor. I mean people may think their color vision is off or something," he chuckled.

"Hey she's *your* wife. She was going for shimmery silver or ironic grey, I think. Not quite there. I'm supposed to come by for her to fix it. The problem is finding the time to do it. If it wasn't for the "having to look professional thing", I kind of like it. Purple is my favorite color. Anyway, what brings you in today?"

"I was in the neighborhood, so I thought I'd stop in to say hi."

"That was nice of you."

"Also, I thought maybe you could look at my eyes?" he asked sheepishly.

"In the neighborhood, huh?" I asked, giving him a suspicious stare. He squirmed under my gaze. "I'm just teasing. Of course I'll look at your eyes. Are you having any specific problems?"

"Vision seems fine. I've just been having some twitching lately. It comes and goes."

"Does your vision move when you get this twitching feeling?"

"Not really."

"Is there any pain, sensitivity to light, redness, discharge?"

"No, to everything."

"Has this been going on for a while, or just recently?"

"It just started a few days ago."

"Does it feel like it's the eyeball moving or the eyelids around it?"

He thought about it. "I guess it's the eyelids."

His vision, pupillary response to light, eye muscle movements were all normal. Then I checked his eye pressures and looked at his ocular structures front to back. Everything appeared normal. Lastly, I fixed the slit lamp light on his eyelids and waited. Eventually, I could see the eyelids twitching.

"There it goes Thi. Did you see it?" he asked anxiously.

"Yes, I saw it. There is a condition called blepharospasm, which is uncontrolled eyelid blinking or twitching. It is a chronic problem which can be troublesome, however knowing a bit more about you and your lifestyle, I think it's more likely just some myokymia."

"What's that?"

"Eyelid twitching."

"Gee thanks doc. I think I could have told you that."

"What I'm saying is, it's harmless and will probably go away on its own. It's usually brought on by fatigue, stress, eye strain. Since your vision is good, I'm going to guess something is stressing you?"

"Yeah," he sighed. "I have been working hard to make sergeant. I've passed all the exams, I have the years in, but I think the captain is looking for me to help solve some open cases before he'll promote me."

"That's doable for you. You're a great police officer. You're very dedicated and good with people."

"Thanks Thi. That's what Lan says too, only she says it louder and has threatened to go talk to my superior for me," he said looking despondent.

"Yikes. Do not tell her where you work. Maybe I can help. Can you tell me something about your case?"

"Well, I don't think I should talk about it with you. You're a civilian."

"I don't need to know names and numbers, just give me the gist of it."

"Okay, I guess it couldn't hurt anything. Who knows, maybe you can help. There was a burglary at this high-end jewelry store. The thief was able to disarm the security system, walk in and clean them out."

"Well sounds like the security system wasn't very good if they could do that."

"On the contrary, they have an elaborate security lock in addition to an alarm and a periodic police drive by. The combination lock is built into the door to prevent bolt cutters from cutting it. The lock needs two combinations. A set of numbers and letters. However, once the combination is made, the lock also requires a key to open it. I mean it's not an eye or fingerprint scanner, but it's pretty good for the average business."

"Indeed. That *is* a high security lock. I didn't know you could get something like that."

"It was custom made. The owner means business, which is probably why they are so determined to catch the thief. There are several security cameras pointed at the door which the thief seemed aware of because he never looked directly at them."

"It's sounding like an inside job."

"Our thoughts as well. However, the owner didn't tell his employees about a secret camera hidden in the sign overhead. It took pictures of the perpetrator from the top, but he was dressed all in black with a scarf over his nose and mouth, so no good physical description of his face. Except there was a moment when he looked up as if trying to remember the combination, so we have a picture of his eyes."

"Are you sure it's a man?"

"Based on height and build, very likely."

"Can I see the pictures?"

"I can bring it up on my computer tablet. It's in my car, I'll go get it."

He disappeared in a hurry and returned in a flash. He brought the image up. It was black and white and a little grainy since it was nighttime. The two best images were of the person with their head down close to the lock and one with the person looking up at the camera. You could see a small light reflex on the eyes. They were evenly spaced and centered.

"Do you have any suspects?"

"A few. There are two female employees who we have eliminated simply because they are too small to fit the size. There are two male employees. One is an older gentleman who's been with them for some time and the other is younger and has only been with them for about a year."

"Do you have photographs of them by chance?"

"Yes, I do as a matter of fact. We took them and put them into their files since they are persons of interest."

He brought up their pictures and showed me. I looked at their physical builds. With the bulky jacket the thief was wearing, it could have been either of them. I zoomed in on their eyes and after scrutinizing them for a while, I handed the computer tablet back to Jaime.

"Well, it's not either of them," I stated decisively.

"Really? How can you be so sure?" he asked surprised.

"The older gentleman has had cataract surgery. You can see the reflection from the implants in his pupils so he would have had to wear some sort of near aid to look at that lock, like glasses or a magnifier especially since it was so dark."

"Oh right. I never thought about that. What about the other guy?"

"He's got an eye turn. It's not big enough to be cosmetically unappealing, but the security image shows your thief without one."

"What? How in the world did you see that?" Jaime asked staring at the image.

"You forget I'm an eye doctor. If you observe the pinpoint of reflected light in his pupils, you'll notice that in one eye it's centered and in the other, it's not. The image of the thief showed that point of light is even in both eyes."

"You're right!" he exclaimed, comparing the pictures of the two people. "I was interrogating that poor soul for hours. He was my most likely suspect. Wow, doc you're good. You probably just cleared two innocent people. But now I've got no suspects and I'm back to square one."

"Hm, tell me about the two women. Perhaps they didn't do it, but maybe they have a partner."

"Seems unlikely. Both are related to the owner. One of them is his niece and the other is his daughter-in-law."

I considered the nature of their relationship to the owner.

"Do you know if the niece has a boyfriend that she may have told the combination to? He could have easily "borrowed" her key if she has access to one."

"As a matter of fact, I did ask her if she was married or had a boyfriend. She stated that she did have a boyfriend."

"This is a longshot, but do you have a picture of him?"

"No, because I didn't figure he would be involved given that she is the owner's niece."

"Understandable, but I have learned in my time dealing with the public that anyone is capable of anything. Maybe he's in her social media pages? Tell me her name and we'll see if she has one."

We searched the various social media accounts on my exam room computer and sure enough, not only did she have a page, but there on her profile picture, was the boyfriend embracing the niece and looking straight into the camera. His build would match, so we zoomed in on his eyes. I noticed something that I hadn't noticed before in the security picture because it was black and white with low contrast. In the social media picture, he had a small, irregular shaped, pigment spot on the white part of his right eye between his iris and nose. I went back to the security picture and zoomed in on that spot.

"Would you mind if I tried to improve the contrast of this image?" I asked Jaime.

"Do what you have to do doc," he replied.

I sharpened the image as much as I could. Then I lightened the brightness and increased the contrast and sure enough, the spot was faint, but it was there. I handed the computer tablet to Jaime with a look of triumph.

"That's your man."

"Are you sure? I need undeniable proof."

"This pigment spot on his right eye," I declared pointing to both images. "Obviously the image quality is not the best on the security image, but the spot is in the same place, same size and shape."

"I'm amazed Thi," he conceded. "I have been working on this for a week. I looked at hours of security tapes of customers. I questioned those two poor employees several times and you solved it in just a few minutes."

"Just lucky?" I suggested, trying to comfort him. "To be fair, sometimes it's better to stand back and look at it from a different viewpoint. Eliminate the negatives you know for sure and consider possibilities. Not every eye disease presents as cleanly as in the textbooks. They may be hidden among other issues. Also, I have seen enough patients in my professional time to understand that sometimes the problem is not just with the patient or in your case suspects, but with the peripherals in their lives. If you can understand the personality of a person and imagine the life of that person, you can imagine their motivations and their actions. Human nature and the human condition if you will. And of course, a little luck is always good."

"I don't know how to thank you. I'm going straight down to the precinct and tell the captain about this. Hopefully it's enough to bring this guy in for questioning."

"I would bring the niece in too. She may or may not be involved, but I suspect she may know something. Perhaps some time in a police station might get her talking."

"I'll do it," he agreed smiling. "I'll have to come here more often when I've got a problem."

"On days like this, I wouldn't mind the company," I said giving him a hug as he headed for the door.

Chapter 3

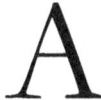driana came into the exam room just as Jaime had left.

"What did Officer Custos want?" she asked bluntly.

"He had some eyelid twitching he wanted to make sure wasn't anything serious."

"And was it?"

"No, very likely stress induced. A case he was worrying about. But I helped him out on both accounts, so it should be better now."

"Uh huh. And did you charge him?"

"What? He's practically my brother-in-law. No, I didn't charge him."

"Dr. Trí if you keep giving away free service, then how are we going to make any money?"

"It was a little thing. I probably wouldn't even know what to charge him."

"He took about 30 minutes. You took his history, examined him, and gave him a diagnosis. Sounds like a level 2 exam at least."

"Oh Adriana," I sighed while avoiding her steely glare. "We'll make it up on the next patients."

"If they ever come in the door. Honestly Dr. Trí, as the office manager I need to inform you that you are running a business, not a charity. Maybe you don't care to get paid, but the rest of us have bills to pay."

"I hear you. I will strive to do better, or at least let you take care of it."

"Hmm. I'll accept that for now, but you're on probation. Anyway, you've had a call from Dr. Moore while you were preoccupied. I think you should call him back. He said something about a business opportunity."

Dr. Chase Moore. He was a classmate of mine from optometry school. He was tall, with luscious dark hair and chiseled features, which I suspect worked in his favor when it came time for grading by many of the female attendings and possibly some male ones too. He spent as much time at the golf course as he did in class, but he still cruised through school thanks to the notetakers. He didn't seem to have many cares in those days, at least financially. His father was a successful optometrist in a well-established practice where Chase was guaranteed to join upon graduation. Not only did he join, but he eventually bought out his father and the businesses next to him and expanded the practice into an enormous multi doctor clinic. It was one of the largest independently owned practices in town. Had I known he would grow into such a force, I might not have opened shop just a few miles from him. I may not have his business acumen, but we usually ended the year with enough money to justify our existence. We also tended to serve the patients that couldn't afford his office anyway. I went to my office and dialed his number. His receptionist answered the phone.

"Good afternoon. See more at Moore Vision Clinic. How can I help you?"

We needed a snappy phone message like this, I thought. "Try us out, at Dr. Trí's eye clinic". Then again, maybe not.

"Uh, yes, this is Dr. Trí just returning Dr. Moore's call. Is he available?"

"Hold on and I'll check."

Even the hold music was a big commercial for his practice. I'm pretty sure the sound of our hold was silence. Gosh, I really wasn't very good at business. Luckily, Dr. Moore picked up before I reached into my emergency stash of comfort treats.

"Dr. Trí. How are you?" he spoke into the phone hurriedly.

"I'm doing great Dr. Moore. I am just getting my lunch break now, so I thought I'd return your call. Can't talk much you know. Next patients will be here soon," I embellished.

"Of course, of course. Every time I drive by your office, I see at least one or two patients in your optical. Business must be good," he replied facetiously.

"What is it that you want Dr. Moore?" I asked dryly, ready to end the conversation.

"Yes, let's get to it. One of my doctors will be out next week for surgery. Instead of taking time to look for a fill in, I thought I'd ask you if you would be interested in helping us out for the week."

I started coughing from the sheer nerve of this guy.

"Excuse me?" I choked out. "You do know that I have a business of my own to look after. Besides, why would I want to work for my competitor?"

"Oh, come now doctor. We both know that my office is at least three times bigger than yours. You've done a respectable job, especially for a cold start, but we also know that you could use the money."

"What are you talking about? We're doing great. I have schedules booked full of my own patients to attend to."

"Uh huh. I had one of my staff call your office and ask for an appointment next week. They said the schedule was wide open."

I opened my appointment schedule on the computer. He was right. A scattering of single appointments throughout the week.

"Well maybe we're not full up yet, but we usually book up during the week. I've got a few appointments scheduled already," I disputed defensively. Why was I trying so hard to impress this guy?

"I'll tell you what. Why don't you move all the patients to first thing in the morning, you can see them and come over to our office after. I'll pay you double the going rate."

"Why would you want to do that? I can't be the only doctor you know," I asked suspiciously.

"True. Okay, look I'll level with you. I meant it when I said you've done well to stay open as long as you have. We have seen a few of your patients and they really like you. They say if their insurance hadn't changed, they'd still be seeing you. So maybe if you try working over here, you might consider closing your office and joining us. We offer excellent benefits."

"Money isn't everything. I have a responsibility to the patients I see that can't afford your prices, not to mention my staff. I also went into business on my own to be my own boss."

"All very good points. However, you know as well as I do that running an optometry practice can be a grind. Let's be frank. You've got the eye doctor part down, but the business part maybe not so much. By joining our office, you would have greater resources. You wouldn't have to worry about paying rent and making payroll. You would only need to focus on the doctoring."

I had to admit he made some good points.

"There's also another thing I would like for you to do while you're here."

"What's that?" I asked ready for the catch.

"I want you to observe my employees. We seem to be short of frame inventory and no one seems to know anything about it."

"How many are you missing? How do you know patients aren't stealing them?"

"Good thought, but we're missing about 10,000 dollars' worth."

"What?" I gasped, choking again.

"Yes, so you can see why I'm ready to pay you a little more to get to the bottom of this."

"Sounds like maybe you should look at your accounting books. Maybe there was an error with the inventory numbers."

"No, I don't think so. I asked for a complete inventory list for the last year from the frame companies so that I could check them myself. Unfortunately, the numbers are real."

"So, you really want me to work at your office to spy on your employees?"

"No, I want you to observe, take data and come up with a diagnosis doctor."

"Why can't you do it?"

"Because I'm too busy trying to run an extremely successful practice and I wouldn't want my staff to think I didn't trust them."

"But won't your staff think something's amiss when a fill-in doctor shows up and starts asking questions and taking notes?"

"Leave it to me. I'll give them instructions to answer any questions you have."

It was a crazy proposition but an intriguing mystery to solve. Then again, I couldn't just leave my office. How would we make money if I wasn't here. Then again, business had been slow, and I could share the money with my staff to boost morale. Dr. Moore took my silence as consideration of his proposal.

"I'll tell you what. Think it over and let me know tomorrow."

"Fair enough. But I must ask, why do you think I can solve this for you when you, who are working there every day, can't?"

"Chet Praxidike," he replied succinctly.

"Excuse me?"

"You know, the first-year student in our optometry class that got thrown out of school for cheating on his optics exam."

"Oh yeah, it's been a while, but I remember him. What's he got to do with this?"

"You were the one that caught him."

"Uh, what do you mean? Dr. Ray caught him and turned him into the dean." I replied nervously.

"No, you alerted Dr. Ray during our optics exam which led to him walking over to Chet and confronting him. He probably would have gotten away with it if it wasn't for you."

"How did you know it was me?"

"I saw you look at Dr. Ray and tilt your head towards Chet. And as Dr. Ray passed by you, he whispered,

"Thanks". I was sitting behind you. I saw and heard the whole thing."

"Um. Okay, maybe I did do those things. But I didn't think Chet would get thrown out of school."

"Dr. Ray takes those tests seriously. He always told us, if you're willing to cheat on an optics exam, you'll probably be willing to cheat on your patients or in business and that has no place in optometry. I'll bet he pushed for Chet to be expelled."

"You're probably right. Just out of curiosity, if you knew, why didn't you tell anyone it was me that busted Chet?"

"Because I didn't want you to have the reputation of a snitch and I agree with Dr. Ray's philosophy. We're a small community. If one optometrist gets busted for illegal or unethical behavior, it puts a stain on us all. What I've been dying to know is how you knew he was cheating. He didn't have any notes on him or in his backpack when they searched it, but I heard Dr. Ray was able to produce the cheat sheet later."

"It was taped on the underside of his desk. He used a shiny, flat metal key chain that was attached to his jeans as a mirror. Dr. Ray suspected that he would try and cheat and asked me to keep an eye out. No one knew."

"I suppose you told Dr. Ray how he did it."

"I did. He appreciated the ingenuity and irony of the situation given it was an optics exam."

We ended our call. Imagine that. Dr. Moore has some moral lines he won't cross. I wouldn't have guessed it. Maybe his proposition wasn't such an insulting offer. I mean he did say I was a good eye doctor, and he respected my office. Well, sort of. The money was very tempting, but how could I tell anyone I was working for a competing business? I was going to have to keep it confidential.

"So, what did Dr. Moore want?" Adriana asked as she strode into my office with the day's mail.

"Believe it or not, he wanted my advice."

"About what?"

"About a challenging case. They involve optical aids. You know, he's good at business, but not necessarily with thinking outside the box when it comes to dealing with unusual situations," I evaded.

"That's true. Did you help him?"

"Not yet. Unfortunately, for his problem, I need to be at his office next week."

"But what about our patients?" she asked.

"I've looked at the schedule. We only have a few that I think we could move to the mornings. He said I could come over after. He'll pay me a consulting fee. I'm still trying to decide on whether to do it or not."

She was silent for a while. I suspect she knew that I wanted to do it. Her expression vacillated from displeasure to resignation.

"Well," she sighed. "I guess the schedule is light enough next week. There are patient orders and insurance fillings we need to catch up on too. I suppose the office will be okay without you for a few days."

"Thanks Adriana. With you steering the ship, we'll stay afloat yet," I smiled.

I drove home that evening full of conflicting emotions. I was happy to have been helpful to Jaime and unsure about if I should help Dr. Moore. I wanted to tell my husband, Fred, about it. However, given our pact to not discuss my office business, I didn't think I should talk to him about it.

An Unconventional Death

I met Fred David Koder while I was a Low Vision Resident and married him a year later. He was not enthusiastic about me starting a practice so soon after graduating. This was understandable since I still had mountains of school loans and limited business experience. I hadn't planned on it either. But when Adriana had approached me about opening an optometry office together, and knowing how practical and hardworking she was, I took the leap of faith.

Adriana Popa and I had met while I was working at a community clinic in Third Ward my first year out of school. Third Ward is an area in the Southern part of Houston with a century's worth of history. It has gone through many periods of economic prosperity and decline as well as cultural changes since its creation. Currently, it is a mix of native Houstonians of all ethnicities and cultures. However, its location close to the center of town puts it in the cross hairs of gentrification. The community clinic we worked at together served the low-income community and there were a lot of Spanish only speaking patients there. I had caught her attention with my attempts at doing an eye exam in Spanish. My Spanish was rudimentary, so my exams consisted of a few Spanish phrases and a lot of hand gestures.

She convinced me that opening a practice together would allow me to be my own boss and she would handle the day-to-day operations of the business. When the lease on our current office space in the Heights area became available, it was such a good deal that I decided it was worth a try. It was a grueling first few years and strained both of our marriages. Although Adriana's marriage didn't survive, Fred respected me enough to let me try. I am thankful that he is gainfully employed in his field of expertise. I know eyeballs, but I confess I didn't know information technology (IT), which is where he excels. Sometimes I get jealous that he can work from home and the only contentious thing he deals with is a computer.

"I'm home," I sang out walking in the door. "I picked up dinner."

"Great," Fred answered from his office with his eyes glued to the computer screen. "I need to work late tonight. We are finishing an update that's going to go live tomorrow."

"Okay," I replied as I came into his office and gave him a kiss on the cheek. "I'll bring your dinner in here. It's General Tso's Chicken from the Chinese restaurant next door to us."

"My favorite. Thanks honey," he said turning his head sideways so as not to take his eyes off the screen.

I lingered for a moment still deciding if I should ask him about Dr. Moore's proposal. Watching him working, I decided it was office related and he was busy, so I left. He turned his head and watched me go, wondering if something was wrong. When I returned with his food, he queried me.

"Everything okay?" he asked, this time facing me when he spoke.

"Yeah, everything's fine. Good luck with your work. I'll see you tomorrow," I smiled and patted his arm before leaving.

It wasn't right to involve Fred when he had his own work to worry about. However, I had to talk about it to someone or I'd start spiraling into an abyss of self-doubt and despair. I decided to call my best friend Lan. She would give it to me straight and she sometimes even had good advice.

An Unconventional Death

From the day we met in elementary school, she was up for whatever I wanted to try. Although I had an older brother and a mother and father, she was an only child and was raised by her mother. Her father had died shortly after the end of the U.S. and Vietnam War. We were both born in the U.S.A. but raised by parents who were part of the wave of Vietnamese refugees to the U.S. after the end of the war. Thankfully we were spared the trauma of war, but we were raised by first generation parents who had real struggles adapting to life in a new country with new customs and a new language to learn. We both grew up relatively poor as our families worked hard to provide better lives for us. With such similar early life experiences, it was no wonder we gravitated towards each other. However, whereas I was more confident in my abilities and about where I wanted to go in my life as a child, she struggled to find her path. This made her shy and more reserved as a child. She was happy to follow my lead. Ironically, as adults our personalities seemed to have switched places. Having to deal with so many confrontational people in my job has led me to retreat more. Fred always knew when I was having a hard time when he would find me sequestered in our guest room quietly engaged in some sort of handmade craft project. I'm particularly fond of the fabric arts. Macrame is under appreciated.

Lan on the other hand, had found her life's passion in cosmetology. She went to beauty school to learn hairdressing, worked for a few years at some high-end salons and finally opened her own salon a few years ago. Success and money allowed her to buy what she wanted. However, without the same financial limitations and likely the stress of running a business, she indulged more on food and drink. Her figure filled out more. If it bothered her, she didn't show it but laughed it off instead. She would often say there was just more of her to love. She blossomed into a strong and confident woman who was not afraid to dress how she wanted, wear her hair and make-up how she wanted and even state her opinions more boldly. That was what attracted Jaime Custos to her.

When I lost my father from complications with diabetes, Lan was there to help me with the loss. We all grieve in our own ways. My brother took some time off work and went on a vacation with his wife. My mom went to church a lot. Lan would come over and tell stories with Fred and me about memorable moments with my dad or just listened when I needed to talk to someone. Likewise, when it was her turn to grieve, I was there for her as well. Jaime came into her life just before her mom was diagnosed with cancer. She tried to push him away, but I told him to be patient with her because of her mom. He showed his devotion to her by remaining steadfast with patience and love when her mom had lost her cancer battle. We were all family now.

Although we had opened our businesses at about the same time, hers was growing quickly while mine was cycling in phases of health and anemia. No doubt her success was due to her unabashed attitude and hair dressing skills. However, she also wasn't afraid to take a chance and embrace trends or try something new even if it seemed far out there, like this rainbow hair dying phenomenon. She didn't restrict herself to the standard blond, brunette, red head variety. Instead, she was one of the first to try all shades of colors. I was usually the reluctant trial run. To be fair, she was my first "patient" in school when we were learning our clinical skills, so I can't complain too much. Second to her cosmetology skill was her business savvy.

An Unconventional Death

Lan built her business within the borders of Montrose, a trendy location frequented by hipsters and artistic people. It has been known as the "heart of Houston" in its early days and was the original center of the LGBTQ community. She had picked a run-down shack on the outskirts of the area, which made it affordable to purchase at the time. She then devoted her time and resources to remodeling it into a fabulous looking, two-story building. Now the area has been gentrified and not affordable to starving artists anymore. However, she was clever enough to build the business on the bottom floor and her home on the top floor giving her a prime location for work and city life. What more can I say? The location was genius, and the salon was fabulous.

I tried a similar approach of picking a site on the north side of the Heights. The Heights area was also undergoing gentrification, so I was hoping that the movement would progress in my direction. Unfortunately, the progression stopped just short of our strip center, and it seems that my area was falling into decline. With half a year left to go on my lease, I was questioning the wisdom of continuing. There were secret whisperings that the government was wanting to expand Interstate 45 in my area, so my fellow tenants and I wondered if our landlord was in talks to cash out on the deal. I hadn't heard much from him about renewing the lease. Alas, another worry line to join my growing collection.

I dialed up Lan's number on my phone as I sat in the kitchen eating my dinner of tofu and pork in brown sauce.

"Hi Thi. What's going on girl?" Lan answered cheerily.

"Hi Lan. You know same old struggle trying to help people see and maybe make a buck too."

"I don't know how you do it girl. If I mess up someone's hair, I just give them a coupon for a free haircut. If you mess up someone's eyes, its lights out. There's no chance of giving them some new eyes."

"You've got that right. Soon you won't have to dye my hair grey, it'll already be there. Anyway, I need to talk to someone about this job I might be taking."

"Are you doing something different at the office. Are you doing Botox too? I've heard of dentists doing that now. If you are, I want the family discount."

"No, I'm not doing anything at *my* office. I was offered a week of fill in at Dr. Moore's office."

"Damn girl. Is business that bad?"

"Sort of, but no. I would be a fill in doctor, but he really wants me to spy on his employees to see who might be stealing eyeglass frames. He says he's lost about 10,000 dollars' worth."

"What the what?" she cried in surprise. "That's a black-market operation going on under his nose."

"Quite possibly," I concurred. "But he has no proof or clue to what's going on. Hence the desperate act of bringing me in to help. It's only a week, so I could be out of the office for that long without too much damage. And he would be paying me very well, so it will make up for it."

"What does Adriana think about it?"

"Uh, I didn't tell her exactly why I would be going there, only that I was going to help out with some optical issues."

"Hmm. What does Fred think?"

"He's working on something for his job, so I don't want to bother him. Besides, this is technically practice related so it's off limits for discussion."

"So, lying to your manager and unable to talk to your husband. No wonder you're a nervous wreck. Yeah, you're very lucky to have me in your life."

"We have established that fact. What do you think I should do?"

"Do you want to do it?"

"I think I could help him, and it would be a break from worrying about my office."

"I'll take that as a yes. Then what are you afraid of?"

"Failure. What if I can't figure it out?"

"Is he still going to pay you for the week?"

"Yes."

"Then you should do it."

"Really?"

"Heck yeah. The guy's not bothering to call the cops about it because he knows they'll never be able to solve it. He can't confront his staff because then they'll get pissed off and quit or sue him for invasion of privacy or some made up crap. You're the only hope he's got. So, he's figured out that some hope of finding an answer is better than no hope at all. Besides, haven't you told me before that he was some stuck up, nepotism doctor that's always making fun of your office?"

"Uh yes."

"Think of it as restitution for your years of mental anguish at his hands. And besides I think you'll solve it. If anyone can, you can."

"Thanks Lan. That's what I needed. I'm going to do it."

"No problem girl. Anytime. Oh, and thanks for helping Jaime today. He told me what you did. That's my girl."

I hung up feeling more secure in my decision. Lan was right. I wasn't a trained detective or anything and Dr. Moore knew that. So, he must have understood that there was no guarantee that I would solve the case. I just hoped I would.

Chapter 4

T he rest of the week went by uneventfully. On the day before I would be starting my "reconnaissance week" at Dr. Moore's office, I was extremely nervous. Perhaps I should have told Adriana the truth. It would have spared me the additional anxiety. I jumped at loud noises and walked around on pins and needles. I could barely make eye contact with her today.

"Are you worried about working with Dr. Moore?" Adriana asked.

"What makes you say that?" I replied sitting in my office and keeping my eyes glued to my computer.

"You've been distracted all day and honestly a little sweaty."

"Maybe a little bit. It's such a big office and I may be a little worried that I won't be able to solve his problem."

"You shouldn't be Dr. Trí," she said gently.

This rare display of sympathy took me so off guard that I looked up at her.

"I shouldn't?" I replied.

"No. I'm sure you'll do great. Maybe I don't say it a lot, but I think you're a great doctor. Always have. That's why I wanted to run an optometry office with you because you're smart, fair, and most importantly, you care about people."

"That's very nice of you to say Adriana. Thank you."

"And while you're there, snoop around his office to see how he runs things. He may be obnoxious, but he's successful so he's doing something right."

"That's a good idea Adriana. I'll do that," I agreed with a smile.

On the day I was starting at Dr. Moore's office, I was ready. I got through my sparse schedule of patients quickly and by late morning, I drove up to Dr. Moore's clinic. The office was massive. It was two stories and was basically its own free-standing building in front of a shopping mall which had a large department store, several boutiques, a fancy bakery, and several nice restaurants. No wonder he was doing well. This was an economic hot spot with several bustling, high-end businesses. There were many cars in the parking lot already. I went in through the front door and up to the reception desk.

"Hello. I'm Dr. Trí," I told the ladies at the front desk. Most of them continued what they were doing. One of the younger staff stopped typing on a computer to acknowledge me.

"Hello, Dr. Trí. You're supposed to go through this door and straight back to the manager's office," she motioned behind her.

"Thank you," I replied cordially and went around the desk and through the door.

The door opened into the optical lab, where a technician was busy cutting lenses for eyeglasses. I walked on through the next door which opened into the break room. There were a few staff members there on the phone or taking an early lunchtime. I kept going until I was finally in a back hallway. Straight ahead led to a backdoor out of the office. To the right were exam rooms and to the left was a staircase that led to the second floor. Under the staircase was a door with the word "manager" written on it. It was an interesting set up to the office. I would think the smell and noise from the optical lab would disperse all around with its central location, but I guess it was closer to the front optical area which was large and curved around most of the front and left side of the office. This made it faster to take patients' finished prescriptions out to them. It's also possible it was in the back when the office was smaller.

I turned left and headed for the manager's office. I knocked on the door.

"Come in," responded a voice from within. I opened the door and went in. It was a small space. There were built-in shelves on the wall but very little furniture. Just a desk with an office chair behind it and a basic wooden chair that faced the desk. No doubt for performance reviews.

"Hello. I'm Dr. Trí. Dr. Moore hired me to fill in for the week. I believe one of your doctors is out for medical reasons."

"Yes, he told me," she said looking me up and down. "I'm Medea. I'm the manager here. I offered to call one of our regular fill-ins, but he said that you could use the money. That was nice of him."

I bit my lip and furrowed my brows trying to stifle my dismay. That louse, I thought, instantly regretting taking this job.

"Yes, nice of him," I repeated with a grimace. "We could all use a little extra cash from time to time you know."

"I do know. When Dr. Chase Moore bought out his father, I was promised to be manager, given my own office and a raise. I did become manager, got my own office and a raise. Unfortunately, with the cost of expanding the building and hiring more staff, it was the last raise I've gotten in years. But you know money isn't everything. I worked for the senior Dr. Moore for 15 years, so when Dr. Chase Moore asked me to stay on, I had to. There's no more employee loyalty anymore, you know?" she lamented.

"Indeed. It must be tough to retain so many employees. How many have you got here?" I asked surprised at her candor to a competitor. I suppose her visual assessment found me harmless.

"We have three opticians, four doctor assistants, two receptionists, a vision therapy technician, a lab technician and four eye doctors. And me of course. I keep the circus going."

"My goodness that is a lot of people," I declared. And a lot of suspects, I thought. "Is everyone full time?"

"For the most part. Everyone gets different days off and some start early and some end late. Scheduling can be a nightmare, especially if someone gets sick or wants to go on vacation."

"What happens when you're out? Is there an assistant manager?"

"I'm never out. I don't really take vacations and I rarely get sick. On the off chance I do have to be out, we triage any problems to the senior staff member in that area. You know, optical problems to the optician, scheduling to reception, etc."

"I see," I said attentively. "Who is responsible for product inventory, like frames and contact lenses."

"I am. I select all the styles. I used to do it for the senior Dr. Moore, so there was no reason to change that. Of course, I delegate labeling the frames and having them put on the boards to the opticians. That way they know where certain frames are that they want to show or sell."

"Makes sense. Who files the insurance?"

"The doctors fill in the exam and diagnosis parts on the computer and the opticians complete the filing after they've made their eyeglass and contact lens orders. If it's only a standard exam, the doctors file it on-line. More complicated medical exams have more insurance requirements, so I'll file it."

"That sounds very efficient. I imagine you keep a tight ship."

"I do." She replied bluntly. "I arrange it so the doctors only need to worry about doctoring. Speaking of which. We have your patient schedule starting after lunch. Dr. Moore wanted you to get acquainted with the office before you're thrown into the deep end."

"That was nice of him," I stated, and I might have meant it if I didn't know the real reason why I was here.

"I'll give you a tour of the office," she said.

She got up from her chair and picked up a headset that had earbuds for listening and a long, thin microphone for speaking into and put it on her head. Then she picked up a small walkie talkie receiver unit and put it in the pocket of her scrubs top and walked past me. I followed her out the door. She pointed out all the exam rooms and explained the color-coded plastic flags on the doorframes that indicated what kind of exam visit the occupant was there for. She showed me the various ophthalmic equipment, which were more abundant and modern than what I had in my little office.

We passed by a staff member whom I recognized because she used to work at my office. She caught sight of me and quickly turned and hurried the other way. So, here is where my former staff end up when they say they've found a bigger opportunity. Why did I agree to do this again?

Medea told me how much time was allotted for each type of exam, which was scanty. She explained the order and flow of the patient experience from check in to check out. She took me upstairs and showed me the storage area where contact lens supplies, eyeglass frames and office inventories were kept. She showed me the vision training room that contained a computer desk station and small chairs around a separate table topped with charts, forms, colored beads on strings, and other training tools. And finally, we arrived at the doctors' offices.

"You'll be using Dr. Smith's office while you're here," she said opening the door and motioning for me to enter.

I looked around. It was a good-sized space. A desk with a computer. A small, armless leather couch with chrome legs sat next to the desk against the wall. I could see myself taking a nap on that. A bookshelf with several eye and medical reference books. A few stacks of industry magazines sat on the desk along with one framed picture of a smiling family.

"Is this Dr. Smith?" I asked looking at the picture.

"Yes. She has beautiful children, doesn't she?" she replied.

"Yes, she does. Has she worked here long?"

"For the past four years. She came on after the senior Dr. Moore sold his part of the office to his son and retired."

"I don't suppose you know what kind of surgery she's having?" I asked casually.

"I believe it's foot surgery."

"And she's only taking a week off to recover?"

"Can't afford to be out longer. If doctors are out, we can't see patients. If we can't see patients, we don't make money."

"I suppose it will be hard for her to go up and down those stairs after surgery. Perhaps you two could switch offices for a while when she gets back."

"Oh no," she uttered firmly. "My office is far too small for a doctor, and I have it just the way I like it. She's young enough. I'm sure she'll recover quickly."

"Probably so," I replied skeptically. I sat down at the desk and opened the bottom desk drawer to put my purse away.

"If there's no other questions, I'll leave you to it."

"I do have a question. I noticed you and the staff wearing those headsets and carrying around walkie talkie units. Is that to keep in communication of each other?"

"Yes. We find it's easier to locate people that way. We used to use the intra office phone line, but people are not always near a phone."

"I hope people don't have it on while they're in the bathroom," I joked.

"You can't hear what someone is saying unless they're pressing the speak button," she replied unamused.

A man walked by and said hello to Medea. She turned and smiled at him. She said something in Greek to him and he nodded.

"Who's that?" I inquired.

"That's Devin, my husband. He does odd jobs around here. He is fixing the door to that storage room. The lock isn't working."

"Is he required to wear scrubs like the rest of the staff?"

"No. We just thought it would be better if he looked like a part of the staff so patients wouldn't be concerned if they saw him around the office from time to time."

"Got it. Good idea."

No sooner had Medea left and I sat down at the desk when Dr. Moore popped into the office.

"Howdy Dr. Trí. About time you showed up for work," he quipped with a sarcastic smirk on his face.

"I had many of my own patients to attend to Dr. Moore," I replied pointedly.

"I assume you've met Medea since you found the office."

"Yes, she seems nice and efficient."

"She's my right-hand man, or woman rather. Been here forever. My dad trained her, so I figured out of respect for the old man, I should keep her."

"If she's that important for the office, why did you give her such a small office on the bottom floor? It's about the size of a closet."

"That's because it was a closet before we retrofitted it into an office. Its better if she's on the main floor so she's closer to the optical and the rest of the staff to troubleshoot when needed. Besides, she's happier there. It's her little kingdom in the office. No one's allowed to go in there when she's not there."

"You mean she locks it? What if she has a patient's order tray or insurance forms or something that someone needs and she's out of the office?"

"First of all, she's rarely out of the office, and if she is, I have a key."

"What do you think of the office?" he asked proudly.

"I'm not going to lie, it's enormous and you have a lot of staff!"

"Yes, and it's still barely enough. If there wasn't such a shortage of trained people, we'd hire more."

"Yes, I saw one of my former doctor's assistants down there. She told me she was going to work for a bigger office, but didn't tell me it was yours," I remarked sourly.

"Oops, you caught me. If it's any consolation, she's very well trained, so good job there."

"That's no kind of consolation at all. And if I were a vindictive person, I would say she was your thief since she clearly lacks good judgement."

"Ha-ha," he laughed and then became serious. "Do you think it's her?"

"No. I mean I don't know yet. I only just got here. I still need to watch everyone's movements and interactions. Other than Medea, your staff seems relatively young. Did they all come on at the same time? Did they all know each other before?"

"As a matter of fact, the opticians did all know each other. They went to school together. I hired one and then he told the others about the office and so we brought them on board. It was lucky too because our previous two opticians retired when my dad did. They didn't seem to like me as much as my dad for some reason."

"I can't imagine why," I replied sarcastically.

"Anyway, it worked out because they are all on the same level and no one can pull seniority. The rest of the staff came on at different times."

"I'm guessing the opticians must get along pretty well if they were already friends."

"Yes, they do thank goodness. It helps morale if they're getting along."

"Do they hang out socially after work?"

"I believe so. They're always whispering to each other and giggling in the office. I would say, they're thick as thieves."

"Interesting choice of words."

"Do you have any other questions about the office or anything before you get started?"

"Yeah, I noticed that there are a lot of patients on my schedule. Is it just because I'm starting in the afternoon?"

"Actually, that's a lighter schedule, since I figured you needed to get used to the office today."

"But that doesn't seem like enough time to spend on the patients. I mean the time you've given me per patient is the time I usually take on their history and preliminary testing."

"Dr. Trí, our doctors' assistants will take their history, do their preliminary testing, and load the phoropter for you. You just need to breeze in, check their spectacle prescriptions and eye health and leave as quickly as you can. Any extra talking is unnecessary chit chat. The more patients you see, the more money is made. I understand you had extra time for talking at your office because you couldn't fill your schedule, but here we move fast. That's why we are so successful."

"But how can you understand your patients' problems without taking the history yourself? And besides, patients appreciate the time. Especially if they have more complicated conditions."

"You're their eye doctor, not their therapist. If they have more complicated problems, then schedule them to come back for another visit. We are a problem focused clinic. If I gave them an hour to tell me their problems, they would have me re-aligning their backs and doing their colonoscopy too."

"But isn't that an inconvenience for them?"

"People must pay for convenience. That's why we also offer our in-house concierge plan. They pay an annual fee, and they can come in whenever they want, we'll fit them in. Besides, people always complain about having to spend a long time at the doctor's office. This way, they can get through their exam quicker."

"So, they're okay with coming in more frequently and paying more for the attention you could have given them with a longer initial exam? That seems crazy."

"That's healthcare in our current times. Now get to work."

I worked frantically to see all the patients on my schedule. It seemed like a whirlwind and one face blurred with another. Thankfully not much unruly behavior to slow me down, although I was constantly having to explain that I was only a fill in doctor and Dr. Smith would be back next week. I observed the staff as they did their work and how they interacted with each other. There were clearly clics, and the newer staff were more ostracized from the others. I wouldn't like such behavior in my office, but then again, we were such a small group so there would be no point to it anyway. Besides, I doubt if Adriana would have allowed it. Here, it seemed that Medea encouraged it. It was almost like each group liked to tattle to her about the others to gain favors. By the end of the day, I was exhausted. I wasn't any closer to discovering the thief, but I did know that this office was no family, just all business.

I got home late that evening. Fred had ordered pizza and had left some in the kitchen for me. I sat down and devoured the first piece in seconds. I was halfway through my second piece when he came in to greet me.

"I didn't hear you come in. You stayed late at the office today," Fred observed with eyebrows peaked.

"Oh yeah. I'm sorry I didn't call to let you know I'd be late. There was this unexpected flurry of patients at the end."

"I was just a little worried, but I'm glad you were busy. That's good for the office."

"Uh, yeah. I guess so," I swallowed hard not feeling good about keeping this assignment from Fred. I didn't like to lie, but I didn't think he'd approve of me working at another office. Especially since he had been so skeptical of me starting my own office at the time. I only had four more days to keep up this charade. I told myself it wouldn't matter in the long run.

"Just shoot me a text next time so I'll know, okay honey?" he asked.

"Of course," I replied. "Actually, I think I might be late the rest of the week."

"Oh, okay. I'm glad business is picking up."

"Yeah, me too," I replied looking down at my pizza to avoid his gaze.

"I'll let you finish your dinner in peace."

"Thanks honey. I'll be turning in early tonight. Got a busy day tomorrow."

"Okay. Then good night," he said and gave me a kiss.

"Good night," I replied, smiling back. Ugh. How was I going to make it through the week?

The next day was just as busy. I found that if I just ignored my instinct to be personable with patients, I could get through the exams more quickly. However, I also noticed a reciprocal amount of aloofness from patients as well. I couldn't worry about it though, I had to make more progress in my reconnaissance.

I happened to be near the front desk when I heard one of the receptionists talking to a patient who mentioned that her insurance had not been filed yet for her last exam. It concerned her because she was getting other medical work done and thought that she had met her deductible. Her insurance said they hadn't gotten the paperwork yet for Dr. Moore's office. I glanced at the patient's file on the computer, there was no information on the insurance filing for the patient, the young lady told her it was sent but was still tied up with the insurance. She said she would contact the insurance company to check the status later. After the patient left, I approached the receptionist.

"I couldn't help but overhear your conversation with that patient. Isn't there a way to check on insurance filings online?" I asked curious to see what she would say.

"I can check on the computer to see if a patient's insurance is entered, but I don't do the filing, so I don't know what their status is."

"Then why did you tell the patient that her insurance had been filed?"

"Because that's what Medea told us to say if patients asked about their insurance."

"I see," I replied.

"*I* could have looked it up for her," the other receptionist said snidely.

"Oh?" I replied. "Are you good at using the office software?"

"Yes. I can look up anything and I'm faster than her too."

"Have you been here longer?"

"By a few months, but I learn fast. Sometimes I even show the doctors how to find things."

"That's very clever of you."

"Yeah, tell Dr. Moore. Maybe he'll give me a raise. My talent is wasted here."

"Does he not pay well?"

"He's not paying me what I'm worth. I even need to stay late to help close sometimes."

"Oh, do you have a key to the office?"

"No, only Dr. Moore and Medea do. But if Medea needs to leave early, there's an emergency key they'll leave for which ever optician could stay to close."

"What do you have to do that they have you stay? Answer phones?"

"No. While they're finishing up with patients, I help put things away and take the trash out. I count the cash payments and the petty cash. If patients are still in the office, I help the opticians clean off frames and put them back on the board. The doctors all leave early of course," she stated giving me a snarky look.

"Yes, well I better go finish my charts before the next patient gets here," I replied eager to end the conversation.

At lunch I caught a break in my schedule. I had a cancellation after lunch which gave me a chance to ask some more questions. I headed to the optical lab to see what I could gather there. The lab technician was busy cutting lenses to be put into eyeglasses.

"Hi there," I greeted him cheerfully. "We haven't formally met. I'm Dr. Trí."

"Hello. I'm 'Doneyet'."

"That's an interesting name. Is it religious in nature?"

"No, that's just what everyone asks me all the time here. 'Are the glasses done yet?'" he joked.

"Oh, right. I get it," I replied chuckling.

"My real name is Chico."

"Well, that's a nicer name anyway. Have you worked here long?"

"For about four years."

"Oh, just like Dr. Smith. Do you like it?"

"It's okay. It pays the bills for now. If they don't give me a raise soon though, I might have to move on."

"Do they know this?"

"No, and I'd appreciate it if you didn't tell them."

"Of course, my lips are sealed. I'm just filling in for the week, so it's not anything to me." I stated nonchalantly. "I know someone who might be interested in doing what you do. How did you hear about the job?"

"Dr. Smith recommended me for it. She knows my mom who told her I needed a job."

"That was lucky. Do you know Dr. Smith very well?"

"Yes. She's a nice lady. She's really the only one that talks to me like a person here. The rest of the staff stick to their little groups and the other doctors don't even know my name. Well, except Dr. Moore since he needs to sign my paychecks."

"That's too bad. You seem like a nice guy. And from what I can see, looks like you do a pretty good job too."

"Thanks. It's okay. It doesn't bother me much. It's just a job you know."

"Yeah, I get it. If you weren't doing this, what would you like to be doing?"

"I got a buddy who's good at restoring cars. He wants to open his own garage customizing cars. He asked me to come work with him when he's got the money for it. I'm trying to save up to invest in the business too. Maybe he'll make me a partner."

"That would be wonderful. Sounds like exciting work and it's always fun to work with friends. I hope it works out for you, Chico."

"Thanks doc. I'd better get back to work."

"Of course," I said and left him to it.

The rest of the day was busy with patients again, but I was forming a list of suspects. There were several disgruntled employees and all of them felt they could be paid more. Of course, in this economy that wasn't too unusual, but was one of them disgruntled enough to steal? They also had opportunity. The clever receptionist was low enough on the totem pole to operate under the radar. She knew how to work the software program and was given leeway to handle frames after hours. Maybe she adjusted the frame inventory in the computer and pocketed a few. Doing this for months or years could add up. Chico, the lab tech wanted more money to start a business with his friend. He also had access to frames. However, it would be difficult to take patients' frames and still fill orders. Finally, all the opticians were friends. They could easily take a frame from time to time. Maybe there was more than one thief. If each one of them took a frame or two it would add up and they could all share in the pot. Like Medea said, employee loyalty was hard to find these days.

I pushed the question to the back of my mind to focus on patients. By the end of the day, I still didn't have a clear answer. As I was walking down the stairs to leave, I bumped into Devin.

"Sorry doc. I didn't see you there," he apologized.

"No damage done," I replied noticing his toolbox. "Still working on the storage door?"

"Yeah, I had to change the lock. Dr. Moore wanted me to. Luckily, I remembered how to do it since I installed the last one too."

"Are you a locksmith?"

"No, I'm just a handyman."

"Are you your own company?'

"No, nothing fancy like that. I used to work sales for a glove company. I drove all around the Houston area on sales calls but got laid off. You know the economy being what it is. My dad did some construction work, so I picked up some things from him and the rest from watching 'how to' videos on the internet."

"Nothing wrong with that. Have a good night," I said cordially.

"Good night doc."

The next day was so busy, I didn't have time to talk to anyone. I just kept my head down and saw patients. As much as my philosophy about patient care differed from Dr. Moore's, he ran an efficient office. They were busy every day. By the end of the fourth day, I was feeling discouraged. I got home to find Fred waiting for me in the kitchen.

"Hi honey. Did you get yourself some dinner yet?" I asked giving him a peck on the cheek.

"I did. There's some Italian food in the fridge for you."

"Thank you. Are you going to sit with me while I eat?"

"If you don't mind."

"Of course not," I said getting my food out and popping it into the microwave.

"So, were you ever going to tell me?" Fred asked a little agitated.

"Tell you what?" I answered nervously.

"That you've been working at Dr. Moore's office this week."

I froze in place.

"How did you know I was working there?" I replied meekly.

"Adriana called. She told me to tell you that tomorrow's morning patients rescheduled, so you could just go straight there instead of stopping by your office. Why didn't you tell me? Is business that bad?"

"Not exactly," I said hanging my head down and feeling the weight of guilt I'd been carrying all week, like Atlas holding up the heavens.

"Then why in the world would you go work for your competition?"

I breathed a heavy sigh. "Dr. Moore asked me to fill in for him while one of his doctors was out. He knew our schedules have been slow lately. He's paying me double the regular fill-in rate. I figured I could share it with the staff."

"That's thoughtful of you I guess but I'm not sure a few extra dollars are a good enough reason to do this."

"Well, there's more to it."

"I'm listening." He was using his serious voice now.

"He is missing about 10,000 dollars' worth of frames and he wants me to figure out who in the office might have taken it."

"Sleuthing! You're there to do sleuthing?" he exclaimed looking none too pleased. "This was why I didn't think you should open your own office. No offense Thi, but you get distracted easily by trying to solve other people's problems."

"Just trying to help a colleague. Thought I could do something good for him and for my staff," I countered weakly.

"You are an eye doctor for goodness' sake. You help people see better every day! Isn't that doing something good? Why isn't it enough?"

"Sometimes it is and sometimes it isn't. I enjoy helping people when I can. Sometimes it's with their eyes and sometimes it's with something else."

"Honey," he said trying to calm down. "You are a people pleaser. People pleasers have trouble saying no, even at their own expense."

"I know I'm a people pleaser, but it's more than that. I kind of like to solve crimes too. You know, stop the bad guys. I'm a 5 ft. 2 in., Asian American woman of average looks and sufficient personality. I didn't get invited to very many parties when I was young. I got picked last for sports teams in school. I had paper and spit wads thrown at me by bullies. But solving crimes, even little ones, usually gained me respect. It even made Lan want to be my best friend," I protested before stopping to gather my composure. Tears welled up in my eyes as I stood by the kitchen counter running my finger around the rim of my water glass.

Fred sat quietly considering my words. The microwave beeped indicating my food was ready. Finally, he stood up and came over to me. He faced me, looked into my eyes, and gave me a big hug.

"I know you had a bit of a rough childhood but you're a beautiful, smart, caring eye doctor now. That should bring you respect, so you don't have to go looking for it anymore."

"You would think. Patients continue to periodically question my credentials and yell at me when I don't tell them what they want to hear. Maybe it's just my ego, but when it happens regularly enough, it can really tear you down."

Fred contemplated my words. "I had no idea that was happening. Listen," he said with intensity. "I love you for all that you are. If you want to work at Dr. Moore's office to solve a crime, you do it. And I know you can do it too because you're clever and dedicated."

"Thanks honey," I replied wiping the tears from my eyes.

"And you know what else?" he asked.

"What?"

"Your food is ready."

"Ugh, you!" I cried giving him a soft jab to the gut.

I sat down hungrily to eat my dinner. Fred sat with me drinking a glass of root beer. We were not big alcohol drinkers. Occasionally we indulged, but not much. We both liked to be clear headed.

"So, have you solved the case yet?" he asked curiously.

"Not entirely. I have a list of suspects. I'll tell you one thing though. Dr. Moore's office may be more successful, but it is like a pit of vipers there. There are clics, people tell on each other, and everyone thinks they deserve more money. They all seem capable of stealing. So, there's motive, but the opportunity to carry something like this out would be difficult. Especially with such a busy office. You think the way they all gossip about each other, that they're watching each other all the time. I wouldn't be surprised if they were all in it together or that they wouldn't think twice about turning each other in for a reward."

"Good point. But if they're not all working together, how could anyone do it alone? That's a lot of frames to steal, so taking it all at once would not go unnoticed."

I stopped just as I was about to put a bite of chicken parmesan in my mouth.

"What is it?" he asked.

"You're right. It would have to be done over time and unnoticed by anyone. I'm pretty sure I know who did it and how. I'll tell Dr. Moore tomorrow. I just hope I'm right."

Chapter 5

I drove directly to Dr. Moore's office the next morning. When I arrived at Moore Vision Center, I went straight to Dr. Moore's office and found him at his computer, drinking coffee and checking his emails. In my excitement from solving the case, I hadn't told Dr. Moore that I would be coming in earlier.

"Dr. Trí, you're here early," Dr. Moore said with surprise.

"My morning patients rescheduled which gives me time to tell you who your culprit is."

"You've figured it out? Fantastic! Lay it on me. Is it one of the opticians?" he asked tilting his head forward and staring expectantly.

"They would seem the most likely, especially since they handle the frames all the time. However, I noticed that they are busy all day and very visible since they are in the front part of the office most of the time. Not enough opportunity."

"Then it's the receptionist, isn't it? She's always asking for more money, and did you see how many tattoos she has? I'm not entirely sure she hasn't been to prison."

"She could be trouble, but no it's not her either. Sure, she's smart enough to know the office computer software and potentially could manipulate the frame inventory, but she complains about doing the smallest of tasks. I doubt she has the motivation and fortitude to do something that would take so much careful time and energy. Besides, she counts the cash at the end of the day. That would be much easier to steal. If she hasn't stolen money yet, as far as you know, then maybe she has ethics or not enough nerve. Who knows."

"She counts the cash! I didn't know she did that," he responded with agitation. "Okay, then who is it?"

"I'm not sure you're going to like this."

"I need to know Dr. Trí. No one is indispensable. Who is the thief?"

"It's Medea."

"What? But she's my right-hand man. She's been here forever. She runs everything here. She's indispensable. How can it be her?"

"It's because she runs everything that it's her. She selects and receives the frame inventory, so she knows exactly what you have and how many. She's in charge, so no one is going to question if they see her with a frame in her hand from time to time and she is always here. Someone who sees her one day may not be there the next so they're not going to give her activities another thought."

"But it's not that she carries around a suitcase. Where is she keeping the frames, how is she getting them out of the office unnoticed? Besides, she's known amongst the frame sales representatives so she can't exactly open shop and sell them out of her house. What would she even do with them?"

"She has a small office room in the back of the clinic under the stairs. It's hidden away from view, and she keeps it locked when she's not there. She's stashing them there until she can take them out of the office."

"But I've never seen her with anything other than her purse, which is not small, but not large either."

"That's because she isn't carrying them out herself. She's got an accomplice."

"But who? One of the other staff?"

"I had thought about that too, but she's the type of person that likes to have dirt on others, not the other way around. No, her accomplice is tied to her until death do them part."

"Devin? But he only comes when there's an odd job to do."

"And what does he bring with him every time he comes for a job wearing scrubs in order to blend in?"

"A toolbox," Dr. Moore announced enlightened.

"Correct. And a rather large one. All your staff wear walkie talkies that lets everyone know where they are at all times for the most part. Medea could easily signal Devin when the coast was clear to just load up the goods and walk quietly out the door. He used to work sales and drove all around Houston. He's sure to know people and places where he can unload stolen frames. I think if you were to go into Medea's office now, you may just find a few frames in her desk drawer."

"But what if you're wrong and I go in there and accuse her without any proof?"

"Considering you're the boss I don't think there's anything wrong with going into an office that's within your business looking for something you lost. I also wouldn't be surprised if you find a few insurance claims that have yet to be filed too."

That last statement poked the bear into action. When there was real money involved, Dr. Moore threw caution to the wind. He flew down the stairs so quickly that I could barely keep up. He didn't even knock on Medea's office door but turned the handle and threw it open. Inside, Medea was sitting at her desk drinking a cup of coffee.

"Can I help you with something Dr. Moore?" she asked surprised by the intrusion.

"Don't mind me, I've lost something, and I think it must be in your drawer. Could you open it please?"

"Why would it be in my drawer? If you tell me what you've lost, I'll be happy to help you find it."

"Open the drawer Medea. I won't ask you again," Dr. Moore ordered, his voice was deadly serious.

She slowly took her key out and opened the drawer. There were the usual desk items. Stapler, post it notes, pens. Dr. Moore turned pale and looked at me. I motioned that he should open the drawer further. He rushed to the desk and took hold of the handle. He pulled it out as far as it would go and there, crammed in the back, were a handful of frames.

"What do we have here?" Dr. Moore asked.

"I was just going to return those," Medea replied without flinching. "They aren't selling well, so the representative said she'll exchange them for us."

Dr. Moore was about to become undone when I cleared my throat. They both looked over at me. I tilted my head to the right and pointed to the floor. Dr. Moore walked over and looked down. There was Devin's toolbox. Dr. Moore leaned down to open it.

"You can't open that, that's my husband's toolbox!" Medea cried.

"Yes, and it's sitting in *my office*," Dr. Moore retorted and flung it open.

We all held our breaths. There inside the box, were about twenty eyeglass cases in the plastic sleeves and boxes that they came in from the frame companies. Dr. Moore picked one up and opened it. Inside were brand new frames.

"And how can you explain this?" Dr. Moore asked as he turned to face Medea.

"I don't have to explain anything. You invaded our privacy. That's an illegal search."

"You're lucky I don't call the police and have them take you out in handcuffs," he replied angrily, but in complete control. "Now give me your office key, pick up your purse and leave right now. You're fired."

"You can't fire me. I've worked here for 20 years. I was here before you even went to optometry school. You wouldn't even know how to run this place. Patients love me. If they find out I'm gone, they'll leave here too."

"It's because you've been with us for so long that I won't prosecute. However, I feel so betrayed by this Medea. How could you? I thought we were family."

"Family?" She exclaimed sarcastically. "Family doesn't stick someone in a closet and only acknowledge them when they need something. Family doesn't overwork someone and not pay them for it. When Devin got laid off, we could barely afford groceries. I asked you for a raise and you kept telling me the office couldn't afford it. But that didn't keep you from getting a new car and a bigger house. So, I didn't steal. I just took what was due to me. Doctor."

"Keys," Dr. Moore demanded holding his hand out.

Medea took them out of the desk drawer lock and put them in Dr. Moore's hand. Then she picked up her purse and held her head high as she walked past us and out the back door. Dr. Moore dissolved into the desk chair.

"I can't believe this," he wailed. "You just never know. How could she have done this?"

"Well, I'm sure this might qualify as kicking you when you're down, but you probably did underpay her. From what I see, she *did* run just about everything around here."

"Maybe," he conceded. "Lesson learned."

"So, you'll pay your next manager better?"

"No, I'll be sure to not let one person run everything. I may even take a few staff off full time and get more part timers."

Boy I really wasn't cut out for business I thought.

"You'd better hop to it, you've got a full schedule of patients to see," Dr. Moore directed after gaining his composure.

"You mean I still need to see patients? I solved the case. There are hundreds of dollars' worth of frames in that toolbox that I saved you. Not to mention the many future frames that would have been stolen."

"Uh, of course you do. What do you think I'm running here, a charity? I appreciate you catching my thief, but I also hired you to see patients. Chop, chop. Get to it."

"Can I at least get my check?" I replied barely able to hide my annoyance.

"I'll put it on your desk, now scoot."

The day was awkward to say the least. Word quickly spread through the office of Medea's firing. The details of the event were not entirely known by the staff but somehow the timing of my last day there seemed to coincide suspiciously with it. Throughout the day, there were looks and whisperings by the staff when I walked by. I never wanted a day to end more. At the end of the day, I was happy to have solved the case, was getting paid and finally able to leave this office for good. My check was sitting on Dr. Smith's desk by the time I was getting my things together. Dr. Moore popped into my office.

"I wanted to say thanks for helping me out," he said seemingly more appreciative.

"Wow, Medea was wrong, you can say thank you," I replied sarcastically.

"I gather you agree with Medea. That had I paid her more, she would have never had to resort to stealing. You probably think I brought this on myself."

"No, of course not. Stealing is stealing and she had no right to do it, but I guess I sympathize with her situation if she wasn't making enough to pay her bills."

"She really could have come to me if she were in such dire straits. Instead, she looked at my new car and house and assumed I was rolling in cash and hording all the money for myself. What she didn't know was that that was the first new car I have had since we graduated from optometry school. And what she didn't bother to understand is that I have a wife and kids and we were living in a small rental house until I could afford to buy us a house big enough to be comfortable. I understand that my success is dependent on having hardworking and competent staff, but you need to understand what it takes to keep an office this big running successfully. We're constantly trying to keep people coming in the door by renovating our space, offering promotions, innovating our services, and upgrading equipment. All these folks have jobs because I take on the risks to keep us growing and ahead of the competition."

"You don't have to justify yourself to me Dr. Moore. Believe me, I am impressed with what you have built here."

"Anyway, I checked all the drawers of Medea's desk. You were right again. She had a stack of insurance claims that she didn't even file. There is at least a year's worth and who knows how many more she might have just thrown away. They were the more complicated medical insurances, so no one noticed because it was her job to file those. It's got to be several thousands of dollars."

"Sorry to hear that, but at least now you know it's probably better to assign that to someone solely dedicated to insurance billing or maybe even an outside company to do it for you. That way when things aren't done, you know exactly who is to blame. Listen to *me* giving *you* business advice. The world has gone mad," I chuckled aloud.

"You're all right Dr. Trí. You're just too busy trying to save everyone to get your hands soiled with the dirty side of business. That's why you should come work with us, you wouldn't have to deal with it, just see patients."

"I thank you for the offer, but I miss my office. Sure, it's not as expansive and successful as yours, but we're a good team and doing good work. See you around."

I left Dr. Moore to ponder the pitfalls of business. I learned a lot in my time at Moore Vision Center. Make sure you know everything that's going on in your office, and value your staff. Additionally, and unexpectedly, I also learned that my prejudices against allotting short exam times may well have been born out of my preferences on how *I* like to conduct my exams rather than on what is necessarily good for patients. The fact that I got through my extensive load of patients each day without necessarily compromising care proved that efficiency does not negate quality. However, it would still be difficult for me to maintain that pace. It's just not the way I like to work and think. If you are stressed and worn out every day you come to work, then what is left for you at the end of the day? A pile of money to medicate your anxiety and sadness.

I went home and hugged Fred. He was delighted that I had solved the case, but mostly that I was done with Dr. Moore's office. A quiet weekend with Fred was what I needed to recharge. So, by Monday, I was excited to get back to work at my practice. I even came in early.

Chapter 6

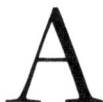

s I walked into my office with my arms full of boxes of delicious treats, I sang out, "Good morning, everyone! I brought doughnuts!"

"Fabulous, I love doughnuts!" John exclaimed excitedly. Everyone congregated in the breakroom.

"I also have a special thank you for all of you for working so hard. I know I was missing in action last week, but I'm back now and I know we'll have our best month yet," I cheered as I handed out envelopes of money to everyone.

Dora, Diya, and John were thrilled and chattered about how they were going to spend their bonuses. I stood apart and swirled my matcha green tea contentedly. Adriana came over and stood next to me so that we were both leaning against the wall and facing the table.

"Thanks Dr. Trí. What an unexpected surprise considering we hadn't seen very many patients lately. Where did you get the money for the bonuses? Did you rob a bank or something?" Adriana probed with a raised eyebrow.

"No, I told you Dr. Moore was paying me well, so I wanted to share with everyone. I appreciate you all. Can't I do something nice without you getting suspicious."

"Of course you can, but let's be real. This is a lot of money for just seeing a few "challenging" patients."

"They were not a few patients. It felt like hundreds," I groused recalling the never-ending stream of people and the accompanying stress.

"You know, I keep my ear to the ground, and I heard some interesting news about Dr. Moore's office."

"Oh. What did you hear?" I asked calmly sipping my tea.

"I heard Dr. Moore fired his manager who had been with him for 20 years."

"You don't say," I replied innocently.

"I wonder why he would do that?" she ruminated suspiciously out loud.

"Maybe she wasn't doing a good job. Or maybe, she liked to question her boss constantly about how to run the office," I quipped.

"No, that's not it. You hold on to good and loyal managers. They're like unicorns." She paused and looked at me for greater effect. "No, I heard that the manager was stealing, which is shocking but not unheard of. The unbelievable part is how she got caught."

"Oh, how did she get caught?" I asked curiously.

"It seems Dr. Moore just went crazy and searched her office and found some stolen frames."

"Wow, that is hard to believe. He always seems so confident and controlled. To just lose it like that? He must have had a good hunch she was up to no good."

"Yeah, or maybe a little bird told him. A bird that was sitting on a nosey *tea tree*," she said vehemently emphasizing the words "tea tree". "That's really why you were working there isn't Dr. Trí?"

"I can neither confirm or deny that accusation on the grounds that it might incriminate me," I replied.

"Why didn't you tell me instead of being so evasive?"

"Because I knew you'd be mad at me for sticking my nose into other people's business when I should be worried about my own."

"Hm yes, I probably would have said something like that. But I'm not so blind or unfeeling that I don't see the abuse you go through with some of these patients. If you need to take some time off to do whatever it is you need to do to recharge, then okay. It's just that most doctors I know go on vacation or go shopping or something. You like to solve crimes."

"I also like crafts. I finished knitting a hat the other day. It's part of a set."

"It's the middle of summer Dr. Trí."

"Exactly. Just in time to be preparing for winter."

"Is it time for patients yet?" she exclaimed, throwing her hands up in exasperation.

The day was a steady stream of relatively healthy patients with no refractive errors. Which means they didn't purchase glasses or contact lenses. It was a nice break from the haggling of trying to convince people they needed something to correct their vision, but it was not good for our bottom line. Soon the happy moods of my staff turned into boredom and worry about the office making money again. The comparison to Dr. Moore's office was stark and a little depressing if I'm honest. So, it was something of a welcome distraction to see my last visitor of the day.

"Officer Custos. How lovely to see you," I called out as Jaime came in the door looking very official dressed in his police uniform.

"Howdy doc. How's your day been?" he replied.

"Uneventful. What can I do for you?"

"And are you going to pay?" Adriana asked, coming out of her office into the optical where we were.

"Well, I'm not actually here for my eyes, I needed to ask Dr. Trí a question. It's a personal issue," he said cautiously.

I suspect he was a little afraid of Adriana.

"Perhaps we should talk in my office," I suggested grabbing Jaime by the wrist and pulling him away from Adriana's penetrating stare.

"What was that stare all about?" he asked once in the safety of my office. "Does she not like me?"

"I wouldn't say that. She's just cranky when I'm not spending my time seeing patients and making the office money."

"Ah, I get it. Is this a bad time?"

"No, it's actually a great time, I just got done with my last patient of the day."

"Perfect. Firstly, I wanted to let you know that we closed that jewelry store case you helped me with a couple of weeks ago. It *was* the boyfriend after all. He cracked when we showed him a blown-up image of his eyes on the security camera. His girlfriend gave him up too. She apparently didn't know what he was planning until after he had done it. After she found out, he convinced her that no one was hurt by the burglary because her uncle had insurance. However, when her uncle confronted her, she spilled everything."

"That's fantastic Jaime. What did your captain think?"

"He thought it was first class police work, which is why I have this," he said pointing to his new sergeant's insignia."

"Congratulations! It looks good on you."

"Thanks Thi. I owe it in part to you. Which brings me to why I'm here. I'm working on a case and wanted your insight."

"Another burglary case?"

"Sort of, but it's more bizarre. A real head scratcher."

"You have piqued my interest. Go on," I urged excitedly.

"There have been reports of things gone missing from several different houses."

"What sort of things? And why wouldn't you simply call it burglaries?"

"Because in some cases it's only one item or a set and the owner can't say when it was taken or that there were any obvious signs of entry into the house, just that the items have vanished. They all have house alarms and some even perimeter security systems which were never triggered."

"Perhaps they misplaced the items and can't remember where they put it. Fred and I do that all the time."

"Yes, I suggested that. But these are very wealthy individuals. They are adamant that the items are so unique and priceless that they have a special place like a display case, mantle or even a safe where the items are kept."

"Have you considered an inside job, like maybe the maid or a cleaning service?"

"Yes, they have all been questioned and cleared. Some of the staff say they were usually not allowed to clean these items because the owners liked to do it or didn't trust them. Some of them didn't even know these items existed because they were kept where they weren't allowed to go, such as in a secret alcove in the closet of the owner's bedroom."

"If the items are so priceless, perhaps the owners haven't really lost them but have hidden them looking for an insurance pay out?"

"I did consider that too which is why I lectured them on the seriousness of fraud and filing a false police report. But they all say it's on the up and up. Besides, when I say these items are 'priceless' some of them may be worth a lot of money, but some are not. They're worth more in sentimental value, which makes them 'priceless' to the owner."

"I see," I replied.

This was a more complicated case. Since it didn't involve eyes, 1 had to admit I was at a loss for ideas. Perhaps I wasn't such a super sleuth after all. I felt a little out of my depth. Perhaps I should quit while I was ahead, and I'm sure Adriana would prefer me focusing on the office more. I could see by the sudden darkness under the door that she was turning out the office lights. Dr. Moore was right, how were we to grow if I didn't start paying more attention to our office. We hadn't updated our website in over a year and our social media accounts were non-existent. I hadn't incorporated new equipment in a few years, and we barely had enough staff. I looked at Jaime's expectant face and I felt overwhelmed and inadequate at the same time.

"I'm sorry Jaime. I'm not sure I can help you with this one. Besides it's late and I'm supposed to have dinner at my mom's house tonight."

He looked disappointed. I hated disappointing people.

"I get it Thi. It's the end of the day, you're tired. This is not an easy case. Could I give you some notes with the particulars? You could look it over at home and maybe something will come to you."

"I don't know if you should be giving me official police papers."

"These are a copy of my personal notes. I figured you would want to chew on it for a while."

I gently sighed and took the papers out of politeness. The expression on my face was probably not encouraging to Jaime.

"Listen Thi. I realize that solving crimes isn't your job, it's mine. But the way you came up with solutions to my last case was amazing. And Lan told me how you helped one of your colleagues solve a problem at his office. You've got a gift. I don't mean just being book smart, which you are, but being able to see what seems like random bits of information and putting them together in a way that the rest of us can't. Like one of those magic eye pictures."

"You mean like a stereo 3D image?"

"Yeah, like how you need to cross your eyes a certain way and stare at a bunch of little dots and shapes to see a hidden picture. Not everyone can do it. Anyway, just thought maybe I'd ask. Have a nice night and say hello to Momma Trí for me."

"I will. Good night, Jaime," I replied and walked him to the door.

Chapter 7

I locked the office after Jaime left. It was amazing how I started the day on a high and ended it feeling low. I got into my car, punched my mother's home address into my GPS device and drove out of the center's parking lot. I knew where my mother's house was since it was the house that we all lived in upon moving to Houston. However, with my mind in the state it was in, I didn't want to risk getting lost. It was admittedly one of my weaknesses. My mind tended to drift to other thoughts while driving which made me miss road signs and the occasional potholes. It didn't help that I was an Asian female. I didn't like adding to the stereotype. GPS maps for driving are one of the best inventions of man, after glasses and contact lenses, in my opinion. I may have a knack for solving crimes, but having someone remind you of when to turn and how much farther your destination was? That was like having an invisible co-pilot. Also, with Texas being such a big state, places were often physically far apart. It seemed no matter where I was going, it would always take at least 30 minutes even without traffic. This gave the mind plenty of time to wander.

It was unusual to gather for dinner at my mother's house during the week, but she told my brother and I that she had an announcement to make. Fred had to work late, so I would be going solo. I dreaded this since Fred was my buffer for dealing with my sister-in-law. Brianna was loud, opinionated, and spoiled thanks to my brother. I turned into the driveway of my mother's house. It was a cute one story, three-bedroom house built on blocks which was how older Houstonian houses were built to deal with flooding. It may have looked old-fashioned, but we never flooded in the time we lived there. It was already filled up with a couple of cars. Everyone was there. I parked, grabbed my purse, and went into the front door.

"About time you got here Thi," Brianna squawked. She had a glass of wine in her hand that resembled a fancy chalice with all the gold rings on her fingers. She was dressed in a very short and fitted dress that might have looked trashy if it weren't a well-cut designer piece that was accessorized with expensive shoes and a stylish headscarf. "We've been waiting for hours. Where have you been?"

"At work," I replied with thinly veiled condescension. "Some of us have to work for a living."

"I work," she retorted. "Today I had to take some phone messages for Vu from clients since his secretary was out sick. And I did a fantastic job didn't I babe."

"Yes dear," Vu replied dutifully and talking to Brianna like she was a toddler. "You did a great job."

"Do you know what this announcement is about?" I asked Vu.

"I don't know for sure, but I have an idea."

"Oh, Thi you're here. Good. Now we can start," my mother announced after coming out of the kitchen and catching sight of me. "I have decided to sell the house."

"What? Why mom?" I asked surprised.

The house may not have been much, but it was always a place of comfort when I needed it.

"Because with your father gone and me getting older, it's too much to keep up on my own," she replied sadly.

"Momma Trí, I agree. You're much too old to be on your own. What if you break a hip or something? Who's going to know and do something about it?" Brianna babbled with mock concern.

"Thank you, Brianna. Have another drink," Mrs. Trí replied flatly.

"Where will you go?" I asked.

"I will be moving in with Vu and Brianna."

Brianna simultaneously spit out some of her wine and choked on it at the same time.

"Is this true Vu?" Brianna asked Vu with daggers in her eyes.

"Yes, babe. Don't worry, we'll set her up in a guest room on the bottom floor of the house. She'll have her own bathroom and access to the garage so she can come and go as she pleases. You'll hardly even know she's there."

"But she'll probably want to use the kitchen for cooking," Brianna protested.

"Do you even know where the kitchen is?" I asked sarcastically since I was sure Brianna didn't know how to boil water.

"I know exactly where it is Thi. It's where we keep the wine," she snapped.

"Mom, you could always move in with Fred and me," I offered.

"Thank you Thi, but your place is too small and too far from where I want to be. Vu lives in a three-story townhouse. It's better for me since it's bigger and I would

79

have room for my special things that remind me of my life with your father. And since his house is on Bellaire, I would be closer to my friends and the Asian markets," she replied.

Our house *was* small and further from the more Asian parts of town, so she was correct on both counts.

"It's a shame you've become so elderly that you feel you can't drive yourself anymore, but you could always use a car riding service to get where you need. And I'm sure Thi and Fred could build an addition for you Mrs. Trí. Their house could use an upgrade," Brianna said deftly managing to insult the three of us in one swoop.

"Brianna, it's already been arranged so there's no point in arguing about it. Don't worry mom, we'll be ready for you whenever you're ready to come," Vu declared definitively.

Whenever Vu took this tone, Brianna knew there was nothing else to be done. He usually gave into her, but when it mattered, he was not afraid to put his foot down. I was grateful for that because my mother would not have wanted to be in a place where she was not wanted.

"So now that everything is settled, let's have some dinner," mom said ushering us into the dining room.

The evening passed amicably enough. Mom, Vu, and I reminisced about life in the house with our dad while Brianna sulked for the rest of the night. By the time I got home, I was back in good spirits.

"Hi honey!" Fred called to me from his office. He was glued to the screen as usual. I was glad he enjoyed his work. "How was dinner?"

"It was good. Mom is selling the house and moving in with Vu and Brianna."

"Really? That's going to be interesting. I hope your mom won't go crazy in the same house as Brianna."

"No kidding. I'm not too worried though. You're talking about a woman who survived war and escaped from her homeland to start over in a foreign country where she didn't speak the language. I'm more worried about Brianna. She may end up drinking even more and dying early from cirrhosis of the liver."

"Funny. By the way, Lan called. Wanted you to call her back when you got in."

"Okay, thanks dear," I replied and headed for the bedroom so I could get out of my work clothes and into something more comfortable. I dialed Lan's phone number, and she picked up after the first ring.

"Hi Thi. How's your mom?" Lan asked between chews of what sounded like chips or carrot sticks. Depending on how tight her clothes were feeling on her at that moment, it could be either.

"Hi Lan. She's well thanks. You need to go see her soon. She's decided to sell her house and move in with Vu."

"What? I love that house. We had such good times there. Does she know that Brianna lives with Vu too?" Lan asked laughing.

"Yes, she does. I think it will be good for her to move in with Vu. Maybe now Brianna won't be spending all his money since mom will be there to monitor her."

"True that. Momma Trí doesn't take flak from anybody."

"How are you doing?" I asked.

"Yeah, I'm good."

"The salon doing well?"

"Yes, in fact I just hired a new hairdresser. He's a bit flamboyant. Likes to wear makeup and shredded clothes but is good with hair. Besides, for my side of town, he fits right in."

"That's true."

"But listen girl, I also wanted to talk to you about Jaime's latest burglary case."

"Not you too," I groaned.

"Now just hear me out. Won't you just look at Jaime's notes and maybe you can see something he didn't consider? This is his first case as a sergeant, so he really wants to solve it. He's been pouring over the details of the crimes every night. It would really mean a lot to him and to me," she pleaded.

"Okay," I acquiesced. "But I can't make any guarantees that I'll find anything. The other cases had aspects that were eye related so maybe I had an advantage. Or maybe I was just lucky. I'm no super sleuth. Maybe I was just looking for a distraction from dealing with the business of my practice."

"I don't think so Thi. Once maybe, but you've solved three cases that I know of. That's got to be more than luck. Don't be so modest. Embrace your talent."

"I've already got a day job. Three cases? Remind me what was the third case?"

"That one in elementary school when that little snot Kimberly Hobart tried to blame me for stealing her pencil case. The teacher was going to call my mom and suspend me if you hadn't outed her as the real culprit."

"The way she treated us then, I was glad to expose her for the lying, troublemaker she was. Just because we were poor, doesn't mean we were thieves. Those rich kids thought they could get away with anything."

"Not when Thi Trí is on the case," Lan cheered.

"Okay, Lan. I'll see what I can do. Tell Jaime to stop by the office tomorrow afternoon."

"Thanks Thi. I owe you one."

I hung up the phone and pulled out Jaime's notes from my bag. All I had to do was approach the case as if I was trying to find a diagnosis for an unknown eye condition, I told myself. First to look at the timeframe. The thefts happened within a few months of each other. Now demographics and social history. All the victims were older males, wealthy and married. At least that was one common thread between them. However, they all worked in different professions such as real estate, finance, oil and gas. One of them was even in politics. Location. They all lived in expensive and exclusive neighborhoods such as River Oaks, Tanglewood and West University (or West U). If it was the same thief or thieves, they sure had a large hunting range. The neighborhoods and houses affected were not immediately close to each other. Not to mention that although the houses in each area were expensive and the neighborhoods exclusive, they had differences in personalities and histories.

River Oaks properties were the most expensive. Houses there sit on sprawling lawns and lush landscaping. It was a shining example of community planning, particularly for a population that wanted to be exclusive. The community was established in the early Twentieth Century by the Hogg brothers. The area's inhabitants are very wealthy, and many are from old money. If you wanted to randomly drive through the area, you would likely be met with suspicion from the homeowners and possibly stopped by security.

The Tanglewood area was developed from brushy fields years later. Unlike River Oaks, it grew organically. As a result, although the neighborhoods are expensive, they are more low-key with many trees. CEOs and top management officials tended to live there, including the late George and Barbara Bush.

For the West U area, property lot sizes are the smallest and number of houses per area size the densest. However, it is the most publicly accessible and active area of the three. Its residents are upper class intellectuals and professionals. Its proximity to Rice University (a private university) and central Houston means a greater population of professors, doctors, architects and the like. Many of the streets are named after authors such as Geoffrey Chaucer, John Dryden, Walt Whitman, and William Shakespeare.

Perhaps they were different crimes that happened coincidently. However, the strange nature of the crimes made this unlikely. These neighborhoods would surely have police or security driving around in the evenings. This would make it difficult for an outside thief to enter without being noticed and if they did break in, why just steal a few items? With such large houses, how would these supposed thieves even know where to look for these items, particularly the ones so hidden away? There were a few items such as artwork and antique jewelry that would have been easier to find, but coin collections, rare books, and even vintage Atari games? Since the items were so disparate, maybe they *were* different thieves. Jaime had made diagrams of the layouts within the houses and marking the locations of where the items were taken. He even noted other objects of worth within proximity that were untouched, such as expensive cars, furnishings, clothing, gold and silver jewelry and décor. He was very methodical and thorough.

He had a map of the city showing all the neighborhoods with the houses affected marked. The burglaries were near the west section of Interstate 610 which is a freeway that loops around central Houston. Tanglewood was west of I-610, River Oaks was east of it, and West U was south of River Oaks. Each area was adjacent to each other, but still far enough away that there didn't seem to offer an obvious connection. The order of occurrence of each burglary also seemed random. It didn't start at one area and stay in that area for a while before moving on to the next neighborhood like a linear, methodical movement, but zig zagged from one place to the next. The order of the incidents reported started in River Oaks, then to West U, then to Tanglewood and back to West U, etc. It was very puzzling indeed. As I stared at the outlines of the neighborhoods on the map, I imagined that it looked familiar to me.

The lines on the map marking the streets in each neighborhood were not all square and linear but snaked around in some areas to follow the bayous that helped with drainage during heavy rain. This made the neighborhoods look less grided and more patchy. It reminded me of smaller blood vessels in the eyes that fanned out to feed the surrounding tissue. The west arm of the I-610 freeway was like the larger vessel from which the smaller vessels branched out. Perhaps the pathology, or crime spree, didn't happen randomly at individual locations but was orchestrated and stemmed from a central source to fan out to these areas. Much like blood leaking at the smaller vessels will show the end stage of the damage, but the problem really starts up stream at the more central, larger vessel. My imagination was running away from me. I had to step away from this healthcare analogy, broaden my view and look at the bigger picture. Not the eyes, but the brain. Human nature. These crimes did not seem to be spur of the moment. Instead, they must have been carefully planned, perhaps by a crime boss who instructed his minions to carry them out.

Maybe another analysis at social history would be enlightening. I read through Jaime's interviews with the victims. They all reported similarly. They noticed one day their item was missing but waited a few days to report it thinking they could find it on their own. Once they determined it was gone, they called the police.

Perhaps one of their wayward children needed cash and sold the items, I thought. However, most of their children were in lucrative professions or prosperous marriages themselves. Additionally, not all of the children were married or lived in town. Another dead end. Then I noticed a little scribble on one of the victims' statement forms. He reported that he had been arguing with his wife when shortly after, he went to his room and noticed his mother's antique wedding ring and other jewelry were missing. That could be something. I'll have to ask him more about it tomorrow.

I fell asleep thinking about the case. By the time Fred came to bed, he had to gather up Jaime's notes, put them away and tuck me in. I dreamt about the case that night. The bits and pieces floated around my subconscious, and I dreamt that I could see the backs of the thieves quietly putting the stolen items into their bags. I could never see the faces of the thieves, but there was something about the bags. My alarm jolted me awake.

"What's the deal with the bags?" I asked myself. "Maybe I'll figure something out today when I talk to Jaime."

Chapter 8

I walked into my office and called out, "Good morning, everyone."

"Good morning," Dora, Diya and John replied from their stations.

"What, no doughnuts?" Adriana asked sarcastically.

"Nope, not today," I replied. "I can't bring it every day. Do you want to get diabetes or something?"

"Not particularly. You know I was just kidding right?" she backtracked.

"Of course."

"Good, because what is no laughing matter is your first patient. First time eye exam and recently diagnosed diabetic. She is complaining of blurred and spotty vision. A1C is in the double digits."

"Yowza!" I uttered. Seems like all my mind energy would be needed for optometry today, but first to modernize the practice. "Dora, are you good with social media?"

"Of course," she replied with youthful confidence.

"Good. Can you set our office up with an account and make the pages cool looking?"

"Sure thing doc."

"Diya, can you email or text some of our recent patients and ask for an internet review for the office?"

"I'm on it, doc," she replied.

"What about me doc?" John asked. "What can I do?"

"Sell more glasses John."

"Uh, okay."

"Sorry, that's all I have for you now. Let's huddle up team," I said motioning for everyone to gather closely. "Hands in." Everyone put their hands in the center of our human circle. "We're going to have a great day today. Let's go Heights Vision Clinic!"

"Heights Vision Clinic!" everyone cried out as we threw our hand out and broke the circle.

"What was that all about?" Adriana whispered to me as the others jauntily returned to their stations.

"Just thought I'd take your advice and start paying more attention to the office."

"Okay Dr. Trí. It's scaring me a little, but I appreciate the effort," she admitted. She picked up her cup of coffee and headed to her office.

I went to my office to put my things away and start the day. The first step was to put on the white coat over my scrubs. Perhaps it was redundant to wear a white coat over scrubs, but I had tried a variety of professional dress until arriving at this current uniform. I initially wore suits or dresses but found patients would often be distracted from their exam by assessing my fashion choices. Then I tried wearing the white coat over my clothes but found it to be too hot. Next, I tried wearing just scrubs which were very comfortable and the dark colors hid stray pen marks and streaks from rubbing against equipment. However, I blended in too much with my staff, and patients had a hard time believing I was the doctor. Which led me to my current uniform of choice, scrubs for comfort, white coat for doctoral legitimacy. I walked into the room to find a middle-aged Latina woman who seemed nervous but pleasant in nature. She was only about 5 feet tall but was decidedly too large for her petite frame.

"Good morning Mrs. Vieja," I addressed her pleasantly. "I understand that this is your first eye exam, yes?"

"Sí, doctora. I don't have any glasses or anything. I can't see very well."

"And how long have you noticed this?"

"For many months now. My sister told me to go to the doctor. I went to the family doctor who examined me and told me I have diabetes and I needed to get my eyes examined, so I came here."

"Very good Mrs. Vieja. You did the right thing," I assured her.

I proceeded to go through the exam, carefully explaining each procedure and what it was for. As we progressed, she seemed to relax more and by the time we finished the exam she was at ease and receptive to my recommendations.

"As you can see in the picture of the back of your eyes, here on your retina there are several areas of bleeding as well as some swelling under the area of the eye that gives you good vision. In addition, you have developed early cataracts, which is the clouding of your eye's natural lens. This is due to your diabetes not being under control. I recommend you be referred to a retina specialist. They are the medical eye doctors and surgeons that can decide if you need laser surgery treatment for your eyes. I will give you a referral form with a list of doctors that are in your insurance and are close by. I will also write a letter back to your diabetes doctor telling her what I have found. After the retina specialist says that you are able, please come back and we will re-check your vision to see if you need any glasses to help you see better, okay?"

"Thank you so much doctora. I feel better now that you have explained everything to me."

"No problem señora. This is what I'm here for. Take care of yourself and think about your health."

I walked her to the front desk and was heading to my office when Diya stopped me.

"Dr. Trí we have an emergency walk in patient. It's a young woman who wears contact lenses and she says her eyes are red and hurt. The next patient is in 15 minutes, do you want to take her?" Diya asked.

"Sure," I replied. "Is she still wearing her contact lenses?"

"I'm not sure and she's not sure. She thinks she took them out, but she said it feels like there's still something in there."

"It could be contact lens overwear or even a corneal ulcer. Did she sleep in them?"

"She said she didn't sleep in them and she never does. She said she takes them out every night and cleans them with contact lens cleaner and throws them away when she's supposed to."

"Hm. Sounds like she's doing everything right. We'll just have to examine her eyes. Put her in an exam room right away," I directed.

Stepping into the exam room I observed the patient. She was a young woman in her early twenties. She was dressed neatly and had her eyes partly closed in discomfort. I looked through her chart to find her name and glanced at her medical and social history.

"Hello Tiffany. I'm Dr. Trí. I hear that your eyes are troubling you. Can you tell me about them?"

"Hi Dr. Trí. Thank you for seeing me right away. Yes, my eyes are hurting me quite a bit and my vision seems blurred. I have been wearing contact lenses for years and I take very good care of them."

"I see. How long have your eyes been feeling this way?"

"Just this morning. It seems to be getting worse as time goes by."

"Okay, let's do a quick check of your vision and then we'll take a look at your eyes and figure out what's wrong," I assured her. I looked at her eyes and could tell she was not wearing her contact lenses. "Do you have glasses?"

"Yes, they're in my purse. Should I put them on?"

"Yes, please do."

She put her glasses on and proceeded to read only to the 20/60 line in each eye. I then instructed her to remove her glasses and looked at her eyes in the slit lamp. Her eyes were red, watery, and sensitive to light. Her corneas were not clear, but slightly opaque and edematous.

"I'm going to put some anesthesia drops and a little 'eye dye' in each eye, okay? It's just a little yellow, fluorescent color that will help me evaluate your anterior corneas better," I told her.

"Whatever you think is best doctor," she responded obligingly.

After application of the fluorescein dye, the anterior structures of her eyes glowed under a blue light and revealed tiny areas of damaged and dead cells across the entire cornea. All signs pointed to a chemical burn.

"Tell me Tiffany, what sort of contact lens cleaner do you use? Is it the all-in-one multipurpose or the peroxide based one with the enzyme disc that fizzes?"

"It's the all-in-one, multipurpose cleaner. I rub the contacts with it and then soak it overnight like I was told."

"That's right. How about the soap you use to wash your hands with? Do you think you might still have had some on your hands when you handled your contact lenses?"

"No, I rinse soap off very well. I don't want them to get on my contact lenses."

"Have you been rubbing your eyes before this all started?"

"Not really."

"Did you use hair spray? Perhaps you may have gotten some in your eyes?"

"I didn't use any hair spray this morning. Why are you asking me all this? What do you think is wrong with my eyes?" she asked, growing fearful.

"Your corneas show damage to the surface that looks like a chemical burn. I'm trying to figure out what you might have gotten in your eyes to cause this. It sounds like you are very hygienic and do a good job of taking care of your contact lenses."

"Yes, I am very careful. I would never handle my contact lenses with dirty fingers."

I was at a loss. According to her appearance and responses she seemed sincere about being clean with her contact lenses, but surely there was something she was not telling me or that I was missing. I smiled at Tiffany as I struggled for an answer and turned to my computer screen to type into her chart. Before I could enter in any information, out of the corner of my eye, I noticed a bottle of hand sanitizer on the desk.

"Tiffany," I said swiveling around in my chair. "This morning, did you use soap to wash your hands or hand sanitizer?"

"I was running late, so I used hand sanitizer," she replied.

"And did you rinse your hands off with water after you used the sanitizer?"

"No. I didn't think you needed to. It's supposed to clean your hands without soap and water, right?"

"Right," I answered slowly. "And after you used the hand sanitizer, did you let it dry before you put your contact lenses in?"

"Um," she hummed trying to think back to the morning's events. "I'm not sure. But my eyes did start to hurt after wearing the contact lenses for about an hour. Did I do something wrong?"

"Well, no and yes. You are right to be vigilant about keeping your hands clean before you touch your contact lenses. However, hand sanitizer is a chemical cleaner. Most have alcohol in them, so you need to let your hands dry or maybe rinse them with some clean water after using them before you touch your contact lenses. This way you can be sure you don't get any on the contacts. Soft contact lenses are like sponges, they will absorb whatever they come into contact with and as you wear them on your eyes, they will transfer this to your eyes too. I believe the chemical burn on your corneas are from the hand sanitizer."

"Oh, my goodness!" she cried with surprise. "Have I ruined my eyes?"

"Nothing some eyedrop medication won't fix. You'll have to stay out of contact lenses until they heal and throw away the ones that you were wearing."

"Of course, doctor. Thank you so much."

I walked her out to the front desk and handed her prescriptions for the medications. We scheduled her for a follow up appointment, and I felt happy that I could solve her problem.

"So, what was wrong with her eyes?" Diya asked.

"She had chemical burns to her corneas from hand sanitizer," I replied succinctly.

"Wow, she didn't tell me she was using hand sanitizer."

"She didn't tell me either, until I asked her, that is."

"How did you think to ask her that?"

"I guess you need to read between the lines sometimes. People tell you things but maybe not everything either because they don't want to or because they don't know that they aren't telling you everything. Sometimes it's because you haven't asked the right question. If you can't get the answers directly from what they say, then you need to think about what they're not saying or what they might be saying. Do you know what I mean?"

"Not really, but that's why you're the doctor," she laughed.

The next patient was already sitting in the exam chair waiting for me in the next exam room. It was an 8-year-old boy who was having trouble in school. He sat fidgeting with the laces on his shoes. He wore a tee shirt with the image of a great white shark on it, mouth open, baring its teeth and ready to take a big bite. His teacher noticed him squinting a lot and having trouble reading, so she sent him to the nurse for a vision screening. He had failed it and therefore was here in my office.

"Hello there Luke. What brings you in today?" I asked casually even though I already knew.

"He failed his vision test at school. I have talked to his teacher, and she thinks glasses might help him with his schoolwork," his mother interrupted.

"I see. How do *you* think you see Luke? Is it hard to see the board at school, or read your books?"

"I guess a little bit. But maybe I'm just not smart enough," he said with downcast eyes and a defeated expression.

"Oh, come now, I don't believe that. You know I heard that sharks don't like to eat people because they taste like chicken. What do you think about that?"

"That's ridiculous. How would a shark even know what a chicken tastes like? They can't go on land and chickens don't live in the ocean," he replied defiantly.

"Well, there you go. That was as smart of an answer as I've ever heard. Let's check your eyes and see if we can't make school easier by seeing better."

I proceeded with his eye exam and he did indeed need glasses. He was near-sighted with astigmatism which would make vision at distance and near blurry and distorted. I put his prescription into a trial frame and adjusted it to his head and eyes.

"Now take a look at the chart across the room. How does that look?"

"Whoa. I can see the letters. Even the smaller ones."

"Yup. Now read me some of this sentence here," I prompted pointing to a simple reading chart. Although he was a little slow, he read all the words correctly. "That sounds great Luke. I think schoolwork is going to be a lot easier now with your new glasses."

"Yeah, I guess so," he replied becoming melancholy.

It seems his initial excitement about seeing clearly had given in to other worries.

"What's the matter?" I asked.

"Kids make fun of kids wearing glasses."

"Are you serious? I think they're probably just jealous that they don't have glasses, besides look at all the awesome people who wear glasses."

"Like who?" he asked skeptically.

"Harry Potter?" I offered.

"He's a kid that got picked on a lot," he replied unconvinced.

"Okay, then how about Superman?"

"Superman doesn't wear glasses."

"Clark Kent does."

"Who's Clark Kent?"

"Clark Kent is Superman's alter ego when he doesn't want you to know he's Superman. He worked as a journalist for a newspaper. Even superheroes want to have normal lives sometimes, right?"

"That's true. Who else wears glasses?"

"What about Iron man? Or the Hulk?"

"Ironman? The Hulk? Are you sure about that?"

"Yes. Whenever Ironman is not flying around shooting bad guys with lasers, he is in his laboratory being a genius. He wears glasses to look at all those computers. When the Hulk is not angry, he is a regular person. He is Bruce Banner, the awesome scientist that wears glasses. It's nothing to be embarrassed about. It just means you want to see clearly so you can use your super brain to be smart."

"That makes sense," he conceded coming around to the idea.

"Luke's mom we've got some great new frames for kids out there. Let's get Luke something stylish so he can conquer the world."

"Thank you doctor," she replied smiling appreciatively.

They went out to the optical and started looking at spectacle frames. I was feeling pretty good about myself. Maybe just being an optometrist was enough for me. I went to Dora's computer and looked at the social media page she had put together.

"That looks good Dora," I told her.

"Thanks Dr. Trí. We should put some promotions on here too."

"That's a great idea. You should get together with Adriana. She may want to feature some specials."

Diya came to get me when the next patient was ready.

"Dr. Trí, the next patient is Ms. Contraire from last week. It's a prescription check, sorry."

I dreaded prescription checks. I spent so much time and attention on my initial testing to ensure the best prescription for patients the first time. It was painful to do it again, especially if the patient was not giving correct responses.

"Did she say what was wrong with her glasses or vision?"

"She said she couldn't see well, and it made her dizzy."

"Did we make her glasses?"

"No, she went to a discount chain."

"Okay, thanks Diya." That was most likely the reason for the discomfort. I don't profess to be the world's best refractionist, but I'm confident in my ability.

"Good morning, Mrs. Contraire. I hope you are well. I understand that your glasses aren't working well."

"Yes Dr. Trí. I picked them up yesterday and they make me dizzy. I can't see a thing. I told the lady that sold them to me, and she told me to try wearing them for a while. I tried for an hour and couldn't do it, so I went back. She then told me that the prescription was probably wrong and that I should go back to the doctor that prescribed them, so here I am."

This was the standard response I often heard from discount chains. They always blamed the doctor.

"Sure, of course we should check to make sure everything is well and there are no changes. What I would first like to do is put the prescription we determined for you in the phoropter to make sure you can see with it," I said while spinning the dials on the phoropter to her spectacle prescription.

I positioned the phoropter in front of Mrs. Contraire's face. I tested each eye individually and then together. She read everything perfectly at the smallest line of 20/20.

"Does this view feel clear and comfortable Mrs. Contraire?" I asked.

"Yes, it looks great."

"Just to be absolutely sure, let me see if you want any adjustments," I said and proceeded to alter the prescription slightly each eye at a time. She rejected any changes. "The prescription is spot on. Let me read the glasses lenses on my lensometer."

I put the glasses in my instrument for measuring lens powers and although the correct powers were present in each lens, the right and left eyes were switched. This was also not an uncommon finding.

"I have found your problem," I declared. "This optical has switched the right and left eye lenses in your glasses. It's no wonder you can't see. The prescription in each of your eyes is different from the other."

"Oh, is that right doctor?" she asked dismayed. "I'm sorry to have bothered you."

"Not at all Mrs. Contraire. That's what we're here for. Take these glasses back to this optical shop and have them re-make the lenses."

"Will they charge me for it?"

"It was their mistake so they shouldn't. I'll write you a note to take with you."

"Thank you, Dr. Trí. I guess I should have bought my glasses here. I just wanted to save a few dollars."

"I can understand that, but as some wise person once said, 'you get what you pay for'."

She left with note in hand and headed out to get her glasses re-made. Luckily, she had an old pair to use in the meantime. It was situations like this that I wished every health insurance company would fully pay for at least one complete pair of eyeglasses to everyone who needed them. Afterall, if you can't see well enough to work and care for yourself, then you can't live properly. I would define that as "medically necessary", but what do I know? I'm just an optometrist trying to help people see better.

I was mulling over this idea when the front door flew open, and a middle-aged Latino man came stomping into the office. He was neatly dressed in a white polo shirt with the collar up, navy blue shorts and white tennis shoes. His hair was combed back and held in place with copious hair product. He was clean shaven and had a deep suntan. He wore a gold watch and a gold signet ring on his pinky.

"I want to get some contact glasses," he demanded to Dora.

"Do you have an appointment?" she asked him.

"Why do I need an appointment? Can't you just sell them to me?"

"You need to have a prescription for them. Have you had an eye exam?"

"No. I have never had an eye exam. My eyes are perfect."

"Then why do you need them sir?"

"Are you mocking me?" he demanded, getting annoyed.

"No sir. But contact lenses are medical devices since you put them in your eyes. You need to be properly fitted for them."

"Hmm. Okay, tell the doctor to see me."

"We have a patient scheduled in 15 minutes, but we may be able to fit you in. Let me check with the doctor, excuse me."

Dora went to talk to me as Diya stayed up front and uncomfortably tried to smile at the man. He made no attempt to be friendly, but instead threw his keys on the counter and pulled out his cell phone to check his social media pages.

"Dr. Trí, there's a man out here that wants an exam for contact lenses. He's not on the schedule and he's never had an eye exam before. You have another patient in 15 minutes. Do you want to see him?"

I really wanted to say no since first time contact lens exams took extra time and I didn't want to be late for the next patient, but then I saw Adriana looking at me from the desk in her office.

"Go ahead and take him in. You can get his insurance card and be checking it while Diya is getting him pre-tested," I told her hoping I wouldn't regret this.

Diya took the man to the pre-testing area and tried to have him fill out the basic office forms with his personal and health information. He squinted at it and then eventually gave up and tossed it back to her saying he couldn't see it well enough to fill out. She started to try and fill it out for him, asking him for the information. I watched the time ticking by and could feel my heart rate increasing. The next patient could walk in at any minute and then I would be late. Nothing made me more anxious than a waiting area full of upset patients glaring at me whenever I came out of an exam room.

"Diya, why don't you go ahead and run him through the instruments, and I'll fill in his information in the exam room," I directed, in an effort to speed up the process.

When the man was seated in an exam room, I stood outside the door and reviewed what information Diya had obtained. He was 45 years old and didn't seem to have any health issues. However, when I saw the autorefractor's reading of his objective refractive error, it showed large amounts of hyperopia or far-sightedness and astigmatism. This was not going to go well I thought. I steeled myself and went into the exam room.

"Hello Mr. Gonzalez. How are you doing today?" I asked pleasantly.

"I'm fine. Are you're the doctor?" He asked looking me up and down.

"Yes, I'm Dr. Trí. Nice to meet you. I understand that you have never had an eye exam before?"

"Yes. I never needed one. My eyes are perfect. My health is perfect," he declared.

"But you are noticing some trouble seeing now?"

"Yes, for some reason I am having trouble reading the street signs when I'm driving and when I'm reading things up close. Someone told me maybe I needed glasses, but I don't want to wear glasses. It doesn't look good. I want contact glasses so I can see everything again."

"I understand. We will need to do an examination of your eyes to find the correct prescription for glasses and contact lenses as well as ensure that your eyes are healthy and able to wear contact lenses."

"Okay, do what you have to do, but I don't want to wear glasses."

"I understand but I must tell you that the initial testing of your refractive error shows that contact lenses will not be as good for your vision as glasses."

"What testing?"

"You know the computer-like instrument that my assistant put your head against where you looked in with your eyes and saw a picture of a barn?"

"Yes."

"That is called an autorefractor. It gives me a starting prescription for your eyes and vision. It shows that you have a lot of hyperopia and astigmatism. This will be very difficult to fit in contact lenses for far and near vision."

"What are you talking about? What's the difference between my far and near vision? A few years ago, I could see everything perfectly."

"Yes, I believe you could. But because you are older now, especially older than 40 years old, your eyes have changed, and you will need two different prescriptions for far and near. Something like a bifocal or multifocal type of lens."

"Are you calling me old? I'm not old. I'm only 45. Look at me. I look very good. My health is perfect. You just need to do your job and fix my eyes."

"Yes sir. I would like to do that, but I must give you all the information about your eyes, so you understand if the contact lenses do not make your vision perfectly clear."

He became quite agitated at this point. His cell phone buzzed and he turned his attention to it. The font size was enlarged on his smart phone, so he was able to read it. He read a text and started to respond to it. I looked at my watch. It was time for the next appointment. I had heard the front door to the office open, so I was sure the next patient was already here.

"Sir, I am going to have to ask you to turn your phone off so we can do the eye exam."

This may well have been the last statement he wanted to hear.

"I don't think I want the eye exam. I came in here to buy contact glasses and all you have done for me is to talk a bunch of talk. You have not helped me at all," he roared.

"But I am trying to help you," I replied to no avail. I could hear the pounding of my heartbeat in my ears at this point. I was sure my face was flushed.

"No! You are not helping me! You are just trying to make me wear glasses!" he shouted, turning red in the face. He was so loud that Adriana opened the door and dashed into the room.

"Excuse me Dr. Trí. Your next scheduled patient is here, so Mr. Gonzalez will have to reschedule," she said with authority and handed him his insurance card.

"No. I do not want to come back here!"

"I'm sorry we couldn't help you. Maybe you can find another office that you will like better," she said motioning to the door so that he would leave.

He got up and stormed out of the room and out of the office.

"Lord have mercy! Thank you for that," I exhaled.

"No problem, Dr. Trí. He was out of line talking to you like that and besides, we don't take his insurance anyway," she pursed her lips and shrugged.

"Thank heavens for small miracles."

The next patient had arrived. She was a woman in her late thirties and had brought her niece as her driver. She reported that she was extremely near-sighted and had lost one of her rigid gas permeable (rgp) contact lenses, so she needed a new pair. With the help of her niece, she filled out our office forms and after completing the pre-testing with Diya, she was seated in an exam room ready for me. Her niece sat in the waiting room.

"Hello Ms. Mallory. How are you today?" I asked as calmly as I could after my last patient.

"I'm good doctor except that I desperately need new contact lenses. I'm very near-sighted."

"I see that you wear rgp contact lenses. We don't see as many people in those these days."

"Yes. I need to wear them since my prescription is so bad."

I looked at the autorefractor reading. Indeed, she was extremely myopic and astigmatic. Her prescription went beyond the parameters of a standard soft contact lens. Rigid gas permeable contact lenses are custom-made contact lenses that are stiffer. This gives them certain qualities that are better for higher refractive errors and eye shapes. Because of their more precise fitting requirements, they must be specially made for each person and often take a week or more to arrive at the office from the manufacturing lab once ordered.

"How long has it been since your last eye exam?" I asked.

"It's been about 5 years."

"That's quite a long time. So were your last pair of contact lenses that old?"

"Actually, they were older. I didn't get a new pair at the last exam. I lost the one yesterday, so I've been getting by on just the one in my right eye."

An evaluation of her remaining contact lens showed it to be very scratched and coated with oils and debris. We proceeded through the eye exam and when we were done, her eye health showed no other issues and the parameters for her new rgp contact lenses were calculated and ready for ordering.

"Ms. Mallory, I have the initial prescription for your new contact lenses. I'll order them from the lab, and they should get here in a week or so. We'll call you when they are ready."

"Okay doctor," she said as we walked out of the room to the front desk. I handed the order form and diagnosis sheet to Dora for her to charge Ms. Mallory and check her out. Ms. Mallory quietly gave Dora a credit card.

"Did you get your new contacts?" Ms. Mallory's niece asked.

"Not yet," Ms. Mallory replied.

"Why not?"

"They have to order them."

"How long will it take to get them?"

"I'm not sure."

"Why don't you give my aunt her contact lenses? Why do you have to order them?" the niece turned to me and demanded.

"Because your aunt wears custom made contact lenses. They need to be made especially for her at the contact lens lab. They should be here in a week or so."

"I don't believe you," she said curtly.

"Excuse me?" I replied taken aback by this statement.

"I said I don't believe you. I think you could give her the contact lenses if you wanted to, but you're purposely keeping them from her," she accused belligerently.

"Why would I do that?" I replied. I could feel my blood pressure rising. "Ms. Mallory, please explain to your niece about these types of contact lenses."

But Ms. Mallory seemed afraid of her niece and didn't want to argue with her. She stayed silent. Adriana came out of her office again with the sound of raised voices.

"You see. She doesn't believe you either, bitch!" the niece shouted at me. Everyone in the office was stunned and silent by this turn of events. Dora and Diya being young looked at me for guidance on what to do.

"There's no need for that type of language," I said as calmly as I could. "I have explained the situation to you. We will put a rush on your aunt's contact lens order and call you when they're ready, so I think it's best you leave now."

"No. I'm not going anywhere until you give me her contact lenses bitch!" she continued to shout defiantly and took a step towards me.

"If you don't leave now, we will be forced to call the police and have you removed from the office," I insisted squaring my shoulders and looking her in the eyes.

"Go ahead I'd like to see you try," she retorted smugly.

Like the answer to my prayer, in walked Officer Custos in full uniform. All eyes turned to him. He stopped and returned our stares.

"Is everything all right?" he asked.

"Officer Custos. This person is refusing to leave our office after being calmly asked to do so. Could you please escort her out?" Adriana entreated him.

He was as surprised as the rest of us at this request, but obligingly walked over to Ms. Mallory's niece.

"Ma'am. These ladies have asked you to leave their office, so you need to do so," he told her calmly.

"They don't have a right to kick me out of here. My aunt is a patient. She just paid them money."

Jaime looked at me and I nodded, but the pained expression on my face told him enough for him to act further. He saw a sign we kept on the front desk counter.

"That may be the case ma'am, but this sign here says that they have a right to refuse service to anyone for any reason. Now you can leave on your own or I can put you in handcuffs and walk you out."

For a moment it seemed like it would come to that, but the seriousness of his countenance and the official appearance of his uniform was enough to make the young woman back down. She and her aunt finally left the office which allowed us all to let out a collective sigh of relief.

"Thank God you came in when you did!" I exclaimed gratefully and frankly on the verge of tears. "Thank you for helping us out."

"No problem. What was that all about?" Jaime asked puzzled.

"Just another unruly patient in the world of eyecare," I replied trying to make light of it and regain my composure.

"She wasn't even the patient!" Dora added.

"It's been a day," I said shaking my head.

"What can we do for you Officer Custos?" Adriana asked him more pleasantly than usual.

"I came to talk with Dr. Trí about something if that's okay?" he replied.

"You don't have another patient for an hour," Dora offered.

Jaime and I looked at Adriana. She threw up her arms.

"Oh, what the hell. After the last couple of hours, we could use some peace and quiet," she acquiesced.

"Thank you!" I sang as Jaime, and I hurried off to my office.

Once the door of my office was closed, I relaxed and took out Jaime's notes from the burglaries case. I spread them out on my desk.

"I've had a look at your notes," I said.

"And what have you found?" he replied.

"A real mystery."

"I was afraid of that. It's hopeless," he sighed disappointed.

"I didn't say that." I replied. "There's always hope."

Chapter 9

I patted Jaime on the arm and effused supportively, "You did a great job taking notes Jaime. Your thinking was organized and methodical."

"Thanks Thi. I appreciate that," Jaime replied pleased.

"It has given us a good starting point. What we need now is just a little more specific information. For example, did the homeowners usually discover the thefts after being away from the house like on vacation or out to dinner?"

"Us?" he asked with a grin. "So, I take it you are going to help me with this case."

"Considering I fell asleep dreaming about it, yes I'd say I'm in."

"Fantastic. With both of our heads together, it's as good as solved," he declared with tempered zeal.

I smiled. Optometry work may have been enough for the wallet, but optometry coupled with unofficial detective consultant work were better for the soul.

"So, are you thinking about the high-end art crime ring in the River Oaks District from years ago where the thieves would monitor wealthy homeowners' social media activity to know when they were on vacation or out for the evening and then burglarize their homes?"

"Yes."

"I considered it too. However, in this case, the homeowners did not report having just been out of town or out for the evening. Seems that the thefts likely happened during the day while they were out to work. The problem is that the domestic workers or spouses were usually at home, and they all reported nothing out of the ordinary."

"There has to be a connection. Were the items stolen a hodgepodge of unique pieces, or were they part of the same era or something like that? Maybe the thieves were catering to a high demand of items for a certain era."

"Let me see," Jaime replied taking out his computer tablet and pulling up a list of the items stolen. "They were all older items for sure."

As he scrolled through the list, his excitement dissipated.

"Well, that was a good thought, but it looks like the items were from different time points. There were some Picasso artworks. Some jewelry from the 1920's era. Signed baseball cards from Babe Ruth to Jackie Robinson. And of course, the Atari games were from what the 1970's, 1980's time?"

"Yes, that seems pretty spread out as far as time periods." I sighed. "May I look at the list?"

"Of course," he replied and handed me his computer tablet.

I scrolled through the list. As I studied the items, I realized that each separate victim's items were all the same types of things. For example, one person only had vintage jewelry taken or only had baseball cards taken. It seems that each house's missing items were collections of treasures instead of a variety of random things from each house. This may have been a matter of convenience since they were probably grouped together in their normal storage places, but maybe not. Then there was that peculiar dream I had about the thief or thieves' bag.

"You sure are thinking intensely Thi. Care to share?" Jaime asked, breaking the silence.

"Almost. Do you know if the Picasso works were paintings or drawings or maybe even sketches? And do you have information on their sizes?"

"I didn't pay much attention to that. I guess I didn't think it was important. Is it?"

"I'm not a hundred percent sure, but I'm working on a hypothesis. I'm thinking they were probably drawings or sketches to make them easier to remove and roll up. Let's see," I stated. I took a deep breath and read the descriptions of the art pieces. "Aha. Yes, in your description it says here original drawings and sketches."

"What does that tell you?" he asked intrigued.

"That these were surely targeted thefts and so the perpetrator or perpetrators must have known that these items were there given their smaller, less flamboyant sizes. Had they been bigger, they may have had a more prominent position in the house. Maybe displayed in large frames. Since these items were relatively small, they could more easily have been taken unnoticed and I'm guessing even fit into a shopping bag, briefcase or even a large purse."

"Good point," he concurred. "So, you're thinking it's definitely an inside job?"

"I'm leaning that way. Do you know if the victims were having marital trouble?"

"Honestly, since it was always the husband reporting the thefts, I don't think I even spoke to the wives beyond a cordial greeting. Some were not even around during questioning and the ones that were, said they didn't know anything."

"How did they seem during questioning? Did they seem nervous?"

"Maybe a little. Come to think of it, they didn't seem to think it was as big a deal as their husbands did. They would usually say the items were insured and considered the matter closed, which is odd because usually you would think they would be worried about the idea of a stranger breaking into their house. Do you think it was the wives?"

"They would have the means and opportunity. We just need to figure out the motive and if they knew each other or were working together. These people are already rich, so I hesitate to think they needed the money, but you never know with rich people. Maybe they were having financial trouble but didn't want to broadcast it so they were trying to recover by quietly selling some things. Is there a way to check into their financial situations?"

"I'll do it and get back to you," he said making notes. After he was done, he noticed that I had pulled up a map of the areas on my computer screen and was studying it closely. "Are you thinking of something else?"

"I was just wondering what's in the area here at the intersection of these neighborhoods. Looks like it might be Richmond St. near I-610 West?" I replied.

"I believe you're right. Do you think that could be the thieves' hideout?" he asked.

"Based on its central location. I think, it's the fixation point."

I zoomed into the map for a street view and moved the position of the street views around looking for a business that all of these homeowners might have frequented, even if they didn't know each other. There was a fancy strip center that had a few cafes and specialty shops in it. Then I noticed on another side, there were several medically related offices. I zoomed in as close as the image would go to see the signage. It was grainy at such a high magnification, but I could just make out a dentist, an Urgent Care Clinic, and a family counseling center. This location made the most sense to me.

I had patients come to my practice from north, west, east and south of my immediate area just because I was the only one that took their insurance, or they worked nearby, or their family lived in the area. Any number of reasons. Hopefully one of which was that I was an awesome eye doctor. My six 5/5-star reviews could back me up on that. Of course, that one, 2/5-star rating was the bane of my existence. Everyone told me it was just a disgruntled person having a bad day and taking it out on me. However, it was enough for me to doubt myself sometimes. Could I do more? Should I do more?

"What more can you do?" Fred would ask me. "I know you. You care about your patients. Don't let one jerk who's upset that you didn't give him a discount ruin your day or erode your confidence."

"I know you're right but I'm sensitive. Maybe too sensitive. It helps me pick up on how people are feeling so that I can adjust my approach, but it also hurts me when those feelings become toxic and are directed at me. Maybe I should hang it all up. Just stop being an optometrist and work at a library or something. Escape to the solitude of my mind," I would reply.

These conversations would happen more than perhaps was healthy. Burnout is a real thing in the healthcare profession. These nights usually ended with me in tears and then I would wake up the next day and carry on.

"There," I decided, pointing to the building's signage. "That medical center. It's possible our victims were all patients at one or all of those offices. Each one of those offices would have access to their addresses and some of their personal information."

"It's a good thought, but there's no way I could enter and ask questions at any of them without a search warrant. And without probable cause, I can't get a warrant."

"Yes, and HIPAA regulations would keep them from telling you if they were even patients."

"Right," he agreed. "It's a good lead, but I don't know how I can follow through on it."

"*You* may not be able to investigate there, but that doesn't mean *I* can't. You know, as a concerned private citizen."

"I can't sanction your involvement in that way. I don't know if it's safe or legal for you to be poking around there. If something goes wrong, I don't know who would bust my butt more, my captain or Fred," he uttered warily.

"It's not like I'm going to be breaking in anywhere. I'll just check them out to see if I might be interested in utilizing their services. By the way, all the victims are married with living spouses, correct?" I queried since one of the businesses was for family counseling.

"Let me confirm," Jaime replied. He pulled up the list of victims and scrolled down their information. "Yes, they are all married with living spouses."

"Excellent. I'll have to block some time in my schedule to go down there. I'll report back to you what I find."

Jaime could see that I would not be deterred. He sighed and voiced his concern again.

"Thi, you're a good friend. But I must tell you, I really don't think this is a good idea and if you get caught, I will need to deny knowing about this."

"Of course," I replied. "I don't intend to get caught. However, you do bring up a good point. To lessen the chances of seeming suspicious, I should probably not go as myself. I should have an alias and maybe a disguise. Lan could probably help me with that."

"Don't go dragging her down there with you. You going by yourself probably won't be so bad, but the two of you is bound to be trouble."

"I only need to borrow an outfit and Lan should probably fix this lavender dream in my hair. I do need a list of the victims' names and addresses for reference. I think you should leave your computer here while you go to the bathroom Jaime. You wouldn't want to get it wet," I instructed him smiling mischievously.

"Why yes, I do have to use the restroom doc. You sure know how to take care of people," he winked and left the room. Plausible deniability was the name of the game.

I pulled out my phone and took pictures of the pertinent information from the case. The names and addresses of all the victims as well as what had been taken from each. I would need this to check their backgrounds and find out a little more about them. The internet is a modern sleuth's best friend. Jaime returned after a bit.

"Are we all done here?" he asked.

"Yup. Stay safe out there, officer," I said dismissing him cheerfully.

"Thanks doc. You do the same. God, I hope I don't regret getting you involved in this case," he lamented shaking his head.

"Me too," I laughed.

Chapter 10

B y the time Jaime left my office, it was almost closing time. I had one more patient that afternoon who thankfully showed up on time and was a straightforward exam for eyeglasses. After finishing up patient care and completing exam charts, I ran a quick search on HCAD for the addresses of the victims. Many of them were longtime residents who probably inherited their homes. Old money. However, one of them was relatively new to the area. It was the man who had his vintage Atari game stolen. Mr. Sunit Ashwar. A quick internet search showed that he made money on software. New money. His wife was Ruchi Ashwar. She looked to be in her mid to late thirties and was very pretty. Her hair and makeup indicated frequent trips to the salon. This could be useful.

It has been my observation that people with "old money" were less open to outsiders than people with "new money". This stems from the fact that people with "old money" tended to know each other through family, connections, or having attended the same schools and social clubs. They were part of a circle that was closed off to outsiders. With this in mind, I figured if I wanted to approach any of the victims for answers in this case, my best bet would be the Ashwars.

The only way to confirm or eliminate evidence to support my hypothesis for this case was to go down to that medical plaza on Richmond and I-610 and get some information. I didn't want to look suspicious or waste time by going into all the offices. Therefore, I decided to target the most plausible one. Looking on their websites, the dentist looked relatively young, so the chances that all the victims were his patients seemed less likely. The older men would likely have an established relationship with a dentist that had been around longer. The urgent care also seemed unlikely. There were bound to be closer locations for each of the victims. Since all the victims had living spouses, I suspected the family counseling office was the best bet.

The exterior of the family counseling office had marble columns and ornate black metal trim. I could tell it was expensive because the sign for the business was written in such a fancy script that it was nearly impossible to read. This was an indication that perhaps they were more interested in appearances than trying to advertise their business to everyone. It was likely that they obtained business from word of mouth as an exclusive and discreet establishment. After all, the whole point of a business sign is for it to be easily seen and read by people. By the looks of the center and neighborhood, I doubt anyone would volunteer information to me looking the way I normally did. A distraught, rich, housewife looking for therapy would better fit the bill. I needed to look the part, so I phoned the one person I knew that liked to shop for designer everything, my sister-in-law Brianna.

Brianna had won the lottery when she married my older brother Vu, a successful lawyer. I guess some might say she was a trophy wife being tall, blond, and well endowed. I found her to be shallow and a bit of a spendthrift. However, she seemed to make my brother happy, so I kept my opinions to myself, most of the time.

My traditional, quiet, Vietnamese parents were shocked when my brother first brought her home. But his undisciplined and reckless behavior before meeting her was threatening to derail his life. He had become depressed in school and dropped out of college. He was drinking heavily and hanging out with the wrong crowd. When he met her in a bar it seemed to change his life. He wanted to impress her and show her that he had a lot to offer. I think he already had much to offer being a good son and brother, but good intentions can't keep you in designer goods. He turned his life around. He worked during the day and went to law school at night. Today, he is a partner in a busy multi-lawyer law firm. I looked up her number on my phone and hoped she was in a good mood.

Ring, ring.

"Hello?" Brianna answered.

"Hi Brianna. How are you doing today?" I asked pleasantly.

"I have had quite the day," she whined unapologetically. "The designer shoes I ordered came in the wrong size. They're way too small for me and now I have to wait for them to send me the right ones."

"That's awful," I replied trying not to sound too condescending. "When you say too small for you, would you say about my size?"

"Hmm, maybe."

"Could you check please?"

"Why?"

"Maybe I could use them if you can't. You usually have such good taste in fashion, I bet I'll love them. And if I can't use them, then I'll be happy to take them back for you," I was spewing lies left and right.

"You could definitely learn something about fashion from me. Fine, I'll go see," she huffed. Good thing she wasn't very bright. She disappeared for a few minutes then got back on the line. "Yes, I think your little, shrunken feet would fit into these."

"Great, I mean I'll tell you what. I can stop by tomorrow morning and pick them up then, okay?"

"Don't you have to work or something?" she asked suspiciously.

"I do, but I don't have any patients scheduled in the morning, so why not stop in to see my favorite sister-in-law?" My nose was growing longer by the second and my pants were about to ignite.

"I am your favorite, aren't I?" she snorted. "I'm not surprised you don't have many patients scheduled. I told you not to open your shop in that area. Not even a decent mall around there."

"My *practice* is doing fine. There are a lot of people who need good eye care in this area," I replied defensively and then reeled it in. Taking a breath, I spoke more calmly. "Anyway, I need to ask you for a favor."

"I knew it. I can't lend you any money. Vu said I could only get one new handbag next week, so my money is already spent."

"I don't need money, but I do need to borrow some clothes tomorrow. I have an appointment near the River Oaks area and I want to blend in. Just for a day."

119

"River Oaks? Are you planning on joining a business there? That would be good because you could sure use a job that pays more," she laughed. "If it's for a career change, I say go for it. This whole eyeglass selling thing is not going to make you rich. You should get a real job like Vu. Of course, I suppose you can't do law with your degree. Maybe he'll let you work in his office filing or something. You know he *is* a partner."

"That's a lovely thought, but I'm going to stick with eyecare for a little longer. Just need to borrow some clothes please?"

"Oh, Okay," she sighed. "I have an outfit that is a little small for me. It's not easy having such a great rack as mine. But don't ruin it and I want it back right away."

"Absolutely. I'll take good care of it. Thank you so much. I'll swing by tomorrow morning." I ended the conversation quickly and hung up to avoid further abuse or suspicion.

I went home and tried to hide my investigative plans from Fred. He's not going to like my getting involved in a criminal case, much less going undercover.

"Hi honey. How was your day?" Fred called out from his office as he was finishing work on his computer.

"Great, I helped a woman with diabetes, a little boy with his first pair of eyeglasses, got yelled at by a mean Latino man and had to have the police remove a patient's belligerent niece from the office. So, you know, a Wednesday," I called back to him.

"That's nice," he replied distractedly and too engrossed in his work to really be listening.

I told him I had some work to do, so I'd eat early and be in our room for the evening. He acknowledged and wished me a good night. I scoured the internet for more personal

120

information on the victims and their spouses. A few of them were successful in their fields with respective industry articles praising their talents. The men that weren't so successful had married wealthy wives. Articles on the wives were usually not found except for an occasional picture and blurb in society magazines at some fundraising function or store opening. I did notice that all the victims had been married to their spouses for some time which challenged my pre-conceived notions that these rich, powerful men often traded in their wives for younger editions every few years. However, some of the wives did seem to have new faces over the years. That's a silent cry for help if I ever saw one. I couldn't even imagine what the lives of these wealthy people were like. Their homes were the size of museum buildings, yet there didn't seem to be more than a handful of people living in them. Maybe it was just true that everything is bigger in Texas.

After a couple of hours on this research I was ready for bed. Before going to sleep, I called Lan. I'd need her to fix my hair before I could go undercover.

The phone rang a couple of times before Lan picked up.

"Thi?" she answered.

"Hi Lan. Have you got a minute?" I asked.

"Sure babe. What's up?"

"Um, well I need to go to a meeting in a high-end part of town and I need to look well put together and rich. I'm going to borrow some clothes from Brianna. Could you help me with my hair and make-up? I don't think lavender highlights screams sophisticated."

"Well, well, well. Where exactly are we going getting so fancied up? You aren't having an affair with a rich, married man, are you?"

"No, of course not."

"Because if you are, does he have a friend?" she laughed heartily.

"I'm going to try and meet with a family therapist on Richmond and I-610. I'm sure they have a lot of high-end clients, so I just want to blend in."

"Are you and Fred having trouble, because I know a therapist that would be a lot cheaper."

"No, we're fine thanks. If you must know, I am looking for evidence of a connection between this family counseling center and burglaries from the surrounding areas."

"Ooh. Does this have to do with Jaime's latest burglary case?"

"Uh, maybe. Probably. Yes. We discussed it when he came by the office today to see if I had any ideas about where to go with it."

"Yea! Thank you for helping him, Thi!" she exclaimed. "I know you'll solve it."

"So will you help me?"

"Sure. Do you want me to come with you? I can play the rich, bored housewife too."

"I have no doubt. If anyone could fool a therapist into thinking you have mental issues it's you, but I'm not sure they are even involved. I think it would be less suspicious if I went alone."

"Thanks, I guess." she replied sounding disappointed and slightly offended. "When do you want to come by?"

"I'll try and get an appointment tomorrow at lunch if I can. I'll swing by your salon before that."

"That will work. Luckily this new hairdresser I've got working for me is good, so I'll have time. See you then."

"See you then, good night."

I wasn't sure what I was going to say or do tomorrow, but I felt compelled to carry it through now. I only hoped my hypothesis was right or else I was risking embarrassment for nothing.

The next morning, I was up early, too pumped up on adrenaline to sleep much. I also needed to swing by my brother's house to pick up Brianna's clothes. I bounded into the kitchen and grabbed a granola bar and a banana.

"Ready to go already?" Fred asked looking at his watch. Unlike me, Fred was an early riser.

"Couldn't sleep. I have a lot to get done."

"I'm happy to hear that business is picking up," he said scanning my face.

"Um, yeah. You know how it is, feast or famine," I replied smiling awkwardly. I should have just grabbed something on the way to the office. I shoved my food into my purse and headed for the door.

"Why in such a hurry?" Fred asked.

"The early bird catches the worm. Have a good day," I remarked kissing him on the cheek and running out the door. I was terrible at hiding things from Fred. I may be good at reading people and situations, but he was good at reading me. So, the less said the better.

Even with the extra stop at Brianna's, I got to the office well before anyone else and checked the patient schedule. I had blocked the schedule an hour before lunch but forgot to block the one after it. Guess I won't be eating lunch today. Probably for the best, Adriana might get suspicious if I block too many time slots. I looked up the number for the family therapy clinic on Richmond and dialed it. I should have practiced acting like a rich housewife, but what did they even sound like?

"Good morning, Richmond Family Therapy," the receptionist answered. "How can I help you?"

"Yes, good morning," I replied in a voice lower than my normal pitch and drawing out my words. "This is Dr., I mean Mrs..." I should have come up with an alias last night. I looked at the picture of our office's grand opening on my desk. Such hopes for happiness and success on our smiling faces. "This is Mrs. Richey, and I would like an appointment with your therapist, Lilith Janus, today at noon."

"Have you seen Ms. Janus before?"

"No, but she comes highly recommended."

"Of course. For new patients I'm afraid I won't have anything for you until next month."

"Next month?" I squeaked. "I mean, I am in a desperate situation now. My husband is thinking about leaving me and I'm at the end of my rope. I can't sleep or eat."

"Perhaps you should contact your personal physician for some sleeping aids," she suggested coolly.

"He won't prescribe me anymore. I must see Ms. Janus. She's the only one that can help me. I've heard it from many of my friends who are her clients." I rattled off women's names from the burglary cases. "Please couldn't you squeeze me in today?"

"Hmm," she considered starting to budge. No comment on the names I dropped which could indicate that they were in fact patients or else she just didn't want to say.

"I'll pay cash," I added.

"Okay, well I guess I could squeeze you in today. Please show up on time. Ms. Janus is very busy."

"I will. See you then," I replied happily as I hung up the phone. "Yes!" I cried and pumped my fists in the air.

"What are you so happy about?" Adriana asked as she stood at my office door.

"Um, well just a personal project I'm working on," I replied casually and closed the tab I had open for the Richmond Family Therapy website.

"Well how about some of that excitement on trying to promote this new frame line and lens options?" she asked.

"Are those the new designer frames?" I asked as I rifled through them.

I loved looking at frames. I didn't consider myself a fashionista, except when it came to eyeglasses. I owned several pairs of spectacles. An inevitable consequence of being in the business.

"They are gorgeous but wow, pretty expensive. Do you think they're right for our patients? People seem to only want to spend enough to cover the basics," I stated as I grabbed a pair of designer sunglasses out and popped them on my face. "I'm going to borrow these just for today."

"You can't make assumptions on what people will buy. We must offer quality goods to show that our office is a quality place. We owe it to people to give them the option. Besides, basic frames will not keep the lights on in this place or keep your employees either," she replied. "You know Dr. Moore is trying to steal John, don't you?"

"Is he really? When is it ever enough for that guy? His practice already has so many employees. And after all I did for him," I bemoaned. "He's going to work himself into the ground to keep them. I know his practice is busy, but I just don't know how he can pay them all."

"By charging higher exam fees, seeing hundreds of patients a week, and selling all high-end products. He doesn't even give them an option for basic. That's probably why we've stayed in business. We get all the patients who can only afford the basics."

125

"Or people who want to see the doctor for more than five minutes," I added sarcastically.

"Sad but true," She replied pursing her lips in quiet frustration. "My cousin's friend went there and swore he only saw the doctor for a minute. It happened so fast he wasn't even sure he saw the doctor except the staff kept telling him he did."

"Why didn't he come here?" I asked feeling a little offended.

"Because he wanted some high-end frames!" she cried throwing her hands up in exasperation.

"Oh," I whispered quietly. "Okay I'll try Adriana."

"That's all I'm asking Dr. Trí," she said. "I know sales is not your thing, but it's a necessary evil."

"You're right as always," I agreed. "I wouldn't have made it this far without you. Nor would I have even wanted to run my own office without you."

"I'm glad we understand each other," she replied pleased with the acknowledgment.

"Um, I need to go on an errand today just before lunch. I blocked off the schedule already."

"Ugh, you're almost as bad as my ex-husband, the lying bastard," she wailed.

"I admit I push the boundaries on promises, but I would hope I'm not as bad as that," I protested.

"No, you're not as bad as that. Sorry. It's just been an awful few weeks."

"What's going on? Something you want to talk about?"

"Not particularly. He was just dragging his feet to sign the divorce papers, but after my constant hounding, he's finally done it. It has taken years and it feels bittersweet, but I can finally move on with my life," she declared with mixed emotions.

"I'm sorry it's been rough for you Adriana. I'm here if you ever want to talk about it."

"Thanks Dr. Trí, but I'm not the sharing type. Anyway, I hope your errand won't take long. We have a few families coming in this afternoon."

"I don't think it will," I said evasively. "Just something I have to do."

"This wouldn't have anything to do with Officer Custos' visit yesterday, would it?"

"Whaaat? Nooo," I stammered nervously like a child caught with contraband candy.

"Uh huh," she replied. She looked out the door of the office. "I believe your first patient is here."

Chapter 11

I finished my morning schedule of patients relatively unscathed. The mom of a 10-year-old boy, who proudly spoke of his achievements on a video game I knew nothing about, held me hostage lamenting over her son's quickly changing spectacle prescription. A lengthy debate over his excessive hours in front of the computer and television screens and lack of outdoor time threatened to make me late for my appointment with Lilith Janus. After counseling them on the current treatment options on myopia control, I scooted them out of the exam room, grabbed my purse, and headed out the door.

"Stay out of trouble doc," Adriana called after me as I shot her a smile.

I sped over to Lan's salon just getting there ahead of the lunch time traffic. There were lots of cars in her parking lot. I'm glad business was good for her. I swung the door open and looked around for Lan. Music was playing, people were chatting, and the whir of a hairdryer made such a cacophony of noise I had to stop for a moment to adjust my hearing.

A tall, medium build man with asymmetrically cut, black and blue hair, pale make up and coal black eyeliner headed towards me. I admired his dedication to fashion as he was wearing black leather pants in the middle of a Houston summer. It was balanced by what might be called a shirt, since it was more like bits of netted black string draped over his upper torso. It probably provided much needed ventilation. He tottered over in platform shoes. It seemed odd to me that he should be wearing such high shoes when he was already quite tall. Then again, compared to me, everyone was tall.

"Can I help you, hon?" he asked me.

"Yes, I'm looking for Lan. My name is Thi. She should be expecting me."

"Oh yes darlin', she did mention you would be by today. I'm Paul, the new hairdresser. But you can call me Ru."

He spoke softly and congenially.

"Nice to meet you Ru," I replied shaking his hand.

"I'll go get Lan," he said as he sashayed across the room to her.

I could see now what the shoes were for. You couldn't walk that way without them.

"Thi!" Lan cried as she bounded over enthusiastically. "Sorry to keep you waiting. I was putting some supplies away."

"No worries," I replied and met her halfway. "Interesting color you've got on your hair. What would you call it?" I asked touching her voluminous, long, and wavy locks.

"Do you like it? It's a mixture of red, blond, and brown highlights. I'm calling it the 'autumn' color mix."

"It's great, only I think your brown is actually orange."

"What?" she asked alarmed. She pulled strands of hair towards her eyes. "Are you sure?"

"Maybe your red and yellow highlights blended together?" I suggested.

"No way. I did each area separately. Are you sure your eyes are not tricking you?"

"I've passed every color vision test we have," I replied holding the orange locks in my hands for closer observation. Then I looked around at the objects in the space and at my hands. "I think it's your lighting. It's distorting the colors of the things under it. Come over to the door and look at your hair in the daylight," I suggested.

We went over to the door, and she looked at her hair.

"Damn girl. You're right," she conceded crestfallen.

"Sorry. It doesn't look bad mixed together with the other colors. Perhaps you could call it pumpkin spice?" I joked.

"Thi!" she exclaimed. "You've done it again. Not only did you find the problem with my lights, but you've come up with a genius marketing vibe. Nothing says autumn more than pumpkin spice."

"Glad I could help. I guess the problem with your lights might have been what led to this as well," I suggested touching the lavender highlights in my hair.

"Yeah, sorry again about that. It would have been cute when we were teens, but I guess not so much now. I promise I'll fix it this weekend."

"You can't fix it now?" I pleaded wondering how I would pull off a rich, housewife persona with it.

"Sorry girl, it's going to take longer than you have time for."

"That's true especially since I was barely able to get an appointment with the therapist at noon so I can't be late.

But how am I supposed to look rich and sophisticated with this hair?"

"I have the perfect solution. I have some wigs."

"Are you talking about the ones that you practiced on in cosmetology school? Because I remember those being pretty hacked up."

"No, those were manikin heads and yes, they were a mess. I bought these wigs to demo to clients who aren't sure if they can pull off certain hairstyles. Kind of like a try before you buy situation."

"That is so smart. No wonder you're so good at business."

"You know it," she agreed with a sassy snap of her fingers.

I followed Lan to her office and changed into the fitted designer suit I had borrowed from Brianna along with a beautiful, silk scarf to tie around my neck. I slipped on the designer shoes she had wanted me to return which made me at least two inches taller. Unlike Ru in his platforms, these shoes made me walk in a stiff, awkward sort of way. It was an extreme contrast to the white coat and comfortable shoes I normally wear to work.

"Rocker chick or Bond girl?" she asked, showing me a couple of wigs. One had short chaotic spikes of hair on top and long locks in the back giving a rocking, mullet vibe. The other wig was a blunt cut, short bob with straight across bangs. A few longer strands framed the face in front and the back had stacked layers for volume and shape.

"I think Bond girl is most appropriate considering I'm going there undercover."

"Good choice," she said and started pinning my hair up to attach the wig. "So which office are you going to again?

The dentist or the therapist?" she asked as she was fixing my make up.

"The therapist. I figured there are dentists spread out all over the three neighborhoods, but only one family counseling center close by. Also, people are more likely to share personal information, such as their home life, what they do all day, how much money they have, with a therapist instead of a dentist."

"Makes sense. How are you going to find out if any of them go there? Aren't there privacy laws or something that prevent you from finding that out?"

"I mentioned the names of the victims' wives when I made the appointment with the receptionist. She didn't acknowledge or confirm anything unfortunately. So yes, it's going to be challenging to get information. And you're right, I couldn't just walk in and ask for their health information as an unofficial consultant for the police. That's why I'm going in as a patient. I should be able to say anything or ask anything I want without suspicion. Now whether they answer me is another story."

"You got balls girl. I may be able to get in with my sass, but I wouldn't know what to say or ask," she admitted.

Her words hit me like a tsunami. A wave of fear washed over me. What if I couldn't figure out what to say either? I could feel my heart rate increasing. Why did I think I could do this? I didn't look like a trophy wife at all. Plain, petite, and practical were how I saw myself. What if the therapist caught on to me? My panic must have shown on my face because Lan's expression changed from jocular to concern.

"Are you okay Thi?" Lan asked.

I swallowed hard.

"I don't know if I can do this. What if the therapist figures out, I'm a fake? I'm not gorgeous or refined. Who's going to believe I'm a rich, trophy wife?"

"Of course, you can do this," she replied looking into my eyes. "Yes, you don't look like a model, but that's why people feel comfortable talking to you and telling you things because they don't feel threatened by you."

"I think that was a compliment."

"Yes, it was. The other reason people feel comfortable telling you things is that you have a way of talking to people that makes them feel heard. Understood. It's a great quality."

"Thanks Lan. But usually, I'm the one doing the analysis. This time I'll be the one being analyzed. How am I supposed to talk with confidence when I don't feel it?"

"I hear you girl. However, when you see this, I think you'll think of yourself as rich, beautiful, and fierce," she proclaimed handing me a mirror and feeling pleased with her work.

I gazed at myself and was shocked at the transformation.

"What do you think?" she asked smiling.

"I think you're a miracle worker," I replied admiring her work in the mirror.

I sure didn't look like a plain egghead now. I wondered what Fred might have thought about it.

As if reading my mind, Lan smiled and said, "Let me know if you want to borrow it for a night out with Fred."

"Maybe after he finds out what I'm up to and gets mad at me," I laughed. "Thanks girl. I'll let you know how it goes."

I gathered up my things, gave Lan a hug and waved at Ru as I walked past him to the front door. He waved out of courtesy but looked bewildered as to who I was. Yes, this disguise will do beautifully.

I arrived about 10 minutes before my appointment to fill out paperwork. The waiting room was lavishly decorated with overstuffed brocade chairs and multiple landscape paintings in ornate gold frames on all the walls. A small bubbling water fountain was nestled in the corner. I detected a scent of lavender in the air. Soothing instrumental music was playing quietly to complete the tranquil environment. An attempt at relaxing all the senses no doubt. This was a good way to get anyone to spill their secrets. The receptionist was walled in behind plexiglass. I approached her as confidently and with as much of an air of wealthy condescension as I could muster.

"Good afternoon. I'm Mrs. Richey. I have an appointment with Lilith Janus at noon," I projected with the same deep voice I used on the phone.

Had *I* heard it on someone looking like me, I would have thought they were hiding something. No time to second guess myself now.

She looked at me with an expression that seemed to say she wasn't impressed. Then she handed me a tablet and asked me to fill in the information. I thanked her and took a seat next to the fountain to fill out the paperwork. I needed the gentle sound of flowing water to calm my nerves.

I noticed they used the same electronic health records software our office had tried. It was cloud based and too complicated for my little office, so we had switched to a more standard in-house network. The form was standard format. It asked for home address, phone number, work information and insurance information. I considered if I should put my home address which was a modest sized single-story bungalow in the heights. It was nice, but not excessive and did I really want them to know where I lived? I remembered one of my old classmates had recently moved into the West University area with her surgeon husband and decided to use that address instead. I skipped the insurance information since I was paying cash and wouldn't have wanted to commit insurance fraud either. On the line that asked what I was coming in for I had to really think about. I wrote "mental anguish" which seemed like an all-encompassing symptom that also told you nothing. I returned the tablet to the receptionist, who took it, and then asked for a fee payment up front.

"But I haven't even seen the doctor yet," I protested.

"That's the office policy. That will be $250 in full," she stated without batting an eye.

"That seems a bit high for a session," I said almost choking on my words as I reached into my purse to get my credit card out.

"Ms. Janus is the best and is fully booked for weeks at a time. I did you a favor by squeezing you in today," she snapped at me.

"Yes, I do appreciate that," I replied handing her my credit card.

After about a few minutes wait, a woman emerged from the inner office looking refreshed like she'd just had a spa day. I recognized her from my background internet searches of the burglary cases. Thank goodness I did my research before I came. She was one of the wives from the River Oaks addresses. Score! That's confirmation of at least one of the victims' connections to this office. She was carrying a large designer handbag. I had always wondered what people with such a large purse could be carrying in there. Today I wondered more than ever.

"Mrs. Richey." A well-coiffed blond woman in a burgundy sheath dress, floral scarf, and neutral heels, called into the waiting room.

"Yes, that's me," I answered as I stood up and approached her.

She looked me over, probably making a psychological analysis based on my appearance.

"This way please," she directed as she motioned for me to follow her.

We went to her office, which was nicely decorated. The tranquil nature theme was carried throughout the office as there were three large, gold framed paintings on the wall of trees in the woods. The painting was very realistic. The frames even seemed to protrude out of the wall as if they were really window casings to another world that I could step into. Perhaps that was her intention by hanging them there, to take the patient's mind out of the bustle of the city and into the serenity of nature. There was a large ornate desk and office chair near a window and in front of it were two plush burgundy salon chairs that faced each other. She took a seat in one and directed me to take a seat opposite her. Her dress matched the color of the chair so perfectly that it was as if she disappeared into it and was only an 'all knowing' head floating on a floral wreath hovering before me. Those steely eyes on an expressionless face peered out at you, ready to extract your deepest insecurities.

"What can I help you with today?" she asked, still gazing at me with piercing grey eyes and a stone-faced expression that revealed nothing.

An internet search into Lilith Janus's background had revealed that she was originally from Pittsburg and had graduated from Brown University with a bachelor's degree in psychology. She earned her master's degree in counseling psychology at Baylor University and had been in the Houston area for the last ten years.

I kept my composure and imagined what these other women would have told her. Funny how it was easier to speak out when I was pretending to be someone other than myself. I suppose it eliminated the need to people please.

"Yes, I got your name from one of my friends, Ruchi Ashwar. She said you were able to help her with the problems she was having with her husband," I began.

I was throwing out a line to see what I could reel in.

"So, you are friends with Mrs. Ashwar?" she asked with an even voice and steady expression.

She's good, I thought. Not admitting to knowing Mrs. Ashwar, but not denying it either.

"Yes, we were relatively new to the West University area when we first moved there and were introduced to each other through mutual friends. We were having lunch one day and talking about how our husbands didn't appreciate us and what we could do about it. Then she mentioned how you had helped her and that I should come see you because you could do the same for me."

"I help a lot of people and each person has their own problems. Why don't you tell me about yours? My receptionist mentioned you were feeling desperate that your husband was going to leave you. Is this correct?" she asked plainly.

"Yes, that is correct," I replied taking out a tissue from my purse and dabbing the outer corners of my eyes. "You see I recently inherited money from my father who's passed away. I am trying to think of a good use for this money, you know like charity or something, but he wants to spend it. We fight about it constantly and he has stormed out of the house several times and stayed out all night. He doesn't tell me where he goes. I think he must be having an affair," I effused with exaggerated emotion.

"Just because he's out all night after a heated argument, what makes you think he's with another woman?"

"Well, I don't have proof exactly. But where else could he be going? Oh sure, he says he's staying at his friend's house, but his friends are married with kids. Would he really be bothering them that much? And lately our sex life has been non-existent. I'm sure I smell perfume on his clothes that's not mine."

She seemed unimpressed with my performance and was scribbling lots of notes on her tablet. I'd better come up with something fast or I could kiss $250 goodbye for nothing.

"When he is ever at home, he is more interested in his collections," I continued.

"What do you mean collections. What kind of collections?" she asked pausing from her notes and leaning her head forward a bit.

"He has sports memorabilia. He owns some signed items from some famous athletes," I concocted. "He has them in display cases. I'm sure they're worth lots of money, but I could care less about them."

"Oh," she muttered pulling back. "Well what type of work does he do?"

"He's a programmer for an oil and gas company," I said instinctively. "Uh, but he's very high up in the company, a manager. He will likely be promoted soon probably to a vice president," I added to sound more impressive.

I sensed I was coming up empty on this fishing trip. Apparently, sports memorabilia wasn't going to cut it. I had to think of something more interesting and quickly.

"Well certainly lack of interest in the bedroom is not uncommon after a few years of marriage and money can certainly cause friction. Perhaps his job is stressful and he's just needing some down time," she concluded sitting back in her chair and her tablet on her lap.

"He also owned several bitcoin shares. He got in early you know, and then sold them before they crashed. He didn't tell me how much money he made, but it must have been a lot because he has been bidding on some NFTs of late. I think he owns a dozen already," I rambled on not really understanding why anyone would want such things.

NFTs are non-fungible tokens. They are data on a digital ledger that certifies that this digital string of information which is used to represent pictures, videos or anything with a digital file is unique and not interchangeable. Kind of like an original Picasso painting versus a print copy, but for the modern computer age.

"Does he?" she asked leaning forward again.

Yes! Back in the game.

"Yes, he goes on and on about how he was one of the first people to start collecting these things and they'll be worth a fortune in a few years. It's like an obsession," I proclaimed.

"Well rare and valuable collections are popular with men of wealth and power. It is a symbol of their strength and sense of status. There's a high you get when you're able to acquire something unique and priceless. Like a type of love, but self-love," she explained betraying a hint of emotion. I was thinking it sounded a little hokey but tell me more good doctor.

"So, are you saying he loves his collections more than me?" I asked with mock indignation.

"Without knowing more about your backgrounds and the history of your relationship I can't say for sure," she backtracked. "It's a possibility that you, as a challenge, have been won. Therefore, the excitement of obtaining a different object of value may be a more appealing use of his energy."

"I'm just an object? Like a trophy? That's awful doctor. I guess what you're saying makes sense. But how can I fix this? If he was having an affair, at least I can confront him and make him pay for his betrayal, but how can I compete with objects?"

"I understand your feelings. They're normal. It's not an easy solution," she counseled sympathetically.

"Oh, then what should I do? Threaten him with divorce if he doesn't pay more attention to me?"

"You could do that if you think the marriage is too far gone."

"I'd like to save the marriage, but what else can I do?"

"Perhaps a more subtle way of getting his attention would be better. Since his collection is very dear to him, perhaps you could take some of the items and put them away for a little while so that he doesn't have them around to distract him so much."

"That's an interesting thought," I replied genuinely intrigued. "But where could I keep them that he wouldn't find them? There isn't a place in the house that he doesn't know about."

"I agree not in the house, they would surely be found. Perhaps you could give them to someone you trust to hold onto for a while."

"I see," I said. "Maybe a family member or friend."

"It would probably be better if it was a neutral party or someone who couldn't tell him where the items were.

Otherwise, he could just retrieve them and then what would you have achieved?"

"Indeed. His loss must be truly and deeply felt so that I can comfort him, and then he can realize how much I mean to him. Is that what you mean doctor?"

"Yes, exactly."

"Oh, and after a while I can restore his treasure to him and be his hero and he would be so grateful to me that he'd never take advantage of me again!" I cried out with zest.

"Well now, I'm not sure that's the best course of action. Perhaps you should consider that in the course of consoling him, you two could reconnect again and he would realize such materials things are not so significant," she said pausing to gauge my level of understanding. "Do you understand what I'm saying?" she asked calmly.

"I think I do," I said slowly, and I did.

Chapter 12

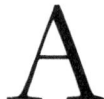

s a healthcare worker myself, I have come to learn
that sometimes it's not as simple as just treating the
symptom of one part of the body as much as also working
with the entire patient.   I often remind myself that I'm not
just working with eyeballs, but with the people they're
attached to.   Spectacles will only help your vision if you
choose to wear them.   Eye infections, from over wearing
contact lenses, can be avoided by simply not sleeping in
them and keeping them clean when they're not in your eyes.
It all seems straightforward, but sometimes patients either
don't have the will or ability to do as they should.   The
problem could be financial, personal (such as busy schedules
or family issues) or psychological.   Understanding what
patients' barriers to treatment are goes a long way in figuring
out how to help them help themselves.   Presenting
treatment in a way that considers the individual's desires
and/or fears can be more effective.

Lilith Janus seems to have found a way to do this while
likely lining her own pockets in the process.   Having a

degree in clinical psychology makes her well trained to manipulate people at their most vulnerable.

Our session time had run out. I thanked Ms. Janus for her insight and made an appointment for another session in a couple of weeks and left the facility. I stopped into the coffee shop in front of my office to change out of my fancy clothes in their bathroom and went back to work. I was happy to have found some insight into the case.

"Successful meeting doc?" Adriana asked as I walked past her, lost in thought.

"Oh, hi Adriana. Yes, I think so," I replied returning to reality.

"I can tell because you're smiling and because your make-up looks fantastic. Not to mention that headpiece. Must have been some lunch date."

I realized I was still wearing the wig and face full of make up when I came into the office. Oops busted.

"Uh, yes well I stopped by to see Lan at lunch. I'm trying out this wig to see if I like this haircut. I think it's a bit too intense for me, don't you think," I jabbered on as I pulled it off my head and headed to my office.

I put the wig on my bookcase and went to the bathroom to scrub my face of the make-up. Didn't want to forget and go home to Fred looking like this. He might think I was walking the street to make rent for the office. The rest of the day went smoothly at work. I phoned Fred to tell him I would be having dinner with Lan tonight and not to wait up for me. After work I stopped by the Galleria Mall to drop off Brianna's shoes and then zipped over to Lan and Jaime's place to share what I had learned.

"How did it go?" Lan asked eagerly.

"Great," I replied excitedly. "I talked with the therapist at Richmond Family Therapy, a Lilith Janus. She wouldn't confirm that Mrs. Ashwar was a patient there, but she didn't deny it either."

"Not sure that gets us anything," Jaime replied discouraged.

"True, but while I was in the waiting room, I saw one of the burglary victim's wives walk out of her office. I recognized her from my internet search of the victims' names. So at least we know for sure that *she* is a patient. That shows a connection between her and at least one of the victims, if not two."

"A coincidence at best," concluded Jaime playing devil's advocate.

"Well how about this. During my appointment time, I convinced Janus that I was a wealthy housewife who is miserable because my husband is more interested in his collection of NFTs than me, and I would do whatever it takes to win his affections back."

"What are NFTs?" Lan interrupted.

"They're non-fungible tokens," I replied.

"And how is that something people want to have?" Jaime added.

"I don't know. Rich people have too much money that they need to invent expensive things to buy, I guess. The point is, she gave me advice on how to deal with it, pretty much cracks the case wide open," I proclaimed dramatically.

"She really believed you were a rich, suffering housewife? That must have been some acting. Especially since you don't exactly look the part," Jaime laughed, then grew serious after seeing Lan's expression. "Uh, no offense Thi."

"Offense taken. I'll have you know with the right clothes and taking more than a minute with my hair and make-up I could be a contender," I declared using my best imitation Marlon Brando voice.

"That's right honey. I loaned her a wig and did her make-up and she looked hot!" Lan exclaimed.

"I'm sorry I missed that," he replied smiling.

"Coupled with some of my finest acting, she didn't suspect a thing," I added.

"Okay, okay. So, what advice did she give you?" Jaime asked, getting back to business.

"Get this. She suggested I pilfer my hubby's precious NFT collection and hide it so that he would not be hung up on such material things. And in his sadness at its loss, he would be emotionally vulnerable and ready to receive and be grateful for my comforting. This would thereby create a situation which would allow me to fill in the hole left by the loss of his precious collection and thus, save our marriage. I think that's what she's told the other women to do, and I'm fairly sure she convinced them to give the valuables to her."

"That is certainly the most unique way of stealing things I've ever heard," Jaime considered. "Have a spouse take it, since they know exactly where it is and when and how to acquire it and no one would even be suspicious of them. Certainly, the staff wouldn't question the activities of the lady of the house. With only a few items taken and covered by insurance, people may not even report it missing."

"Precisely. Who knows how long she's been doing it or with how many people? However, it seems she eventually found unwitting accomplices that took items worth too much sentimentally to the victims to just be forgotten. Therefore, husbands reported them stolen hoping they could be found," I concluded.

"It's an interesting theory, but without hard evidence it's still only a theory. Telling a judge, "I think" and "fairly sure", will not get me a search warrant," Jaime stated. "And where would I even search? Would she be storing them in a warehouse or passing the items off to another person?"

"Yes, I haven't worked all of that out yet, but having at least one of the victim's wives as a patient is evidence of a connection. Isn't that enough to bring her in for questioning?" I asked naively. "Maybe bringing her to a police station and putting the screws to her would prompt her to confess."

"Maybe in the cop shows Thi, but this is real life. If anything, she'd slap the department with a harassment lawsuit. Sounds like she's only suggesting a course of action without explicitly telling you to do it. It's not strong enough."

"What would be strong enough evidence?" I asked.

"A confession by Ms. Janus of course. Possession of the physical items stolen. Testimony from the victims," Jaime rattled off.

"How about admission from one of the wives that she took the stolen items at Ms. Janus's suggestion and maybe even that she gave the items to Ms. Janus?" I queried. "Would that work?"

"Sure. But if this therapist is as good at manipulating people as you say, I doubt you'll be able to find one of them to betray her," he replied.

"Maybe so, but nothing ventured, nothing gained as the saying goes."

"Thi, I appreciate your help, but don't be getting in over your head. Leave it to the law enforcement officials. I'll try asking my captain for permission to surveillance Ms. Janus's office. So, let's agree to that and put an end to the matter. Promise me Thi."

"I promise to leave it to you to surveil Ms. Janus's office," I agreed.

146

I changed the subject and began talking about chick flick movies, shopping, and make-up. This achieved its desired effect as Jaime excused himself with the pretext of needing to go to bed early and he soon left us on our own.

"Okay, now that you have successfully gotten rid of my husband, what are you really planning to do?" Lan asked mischievously.

"Oh, you know me so well. I'm thinking we need to get one of those wives to talk," I stated, rattling the ice in my glass and sipping my drink.

"How are you going to do that? Rich people don't like to talk to people outside their circle. Playing dress up isn't going to fool them. They know each other," she replied.

"True. But one of them is new to their circle. Mrs. Ashwar of West University. She's several years younger than the others and isn't in any pictures of their societal occasions. I noticed in her on-line pictures that she enjoys nice haircuts and manicures. Sooo, I was thinking we could get her to come to your salon and spill the dirt."

"I should have known I'd get pulled into this," she laughed.

"Uh, as I recall, you were the one begging me to help. I was more or less happy doing eye exams on the wrong side of town," I pointed out.

"Okay, okay. You're right. I brought it on myself. She probably has her own hairdresser though. Why would she come to my salon, even if it is the best?"

"If there's one thing I know about rich people, they can be pretty cheap on the day-to-day expenses. They like to look rich without spending money so maybe a free haircut and manicure special would entice her to your place."

"I refuse to give her a free haircut. A free shampoo and blow out is the best you'll get. And you know I don't do

147

manicures," Lan said with a sour expression. "My salon is classy, and I don't want to contribute to stereotypes about Vietnamese ladies doing nails."

"But that's what will be so convincing. We're Vietnamese Americans, so she won't think anything about us doing her nails. She might not even think we speak much English, so she won't think anything about talking in front of us."

"And by us doing nails, do you mean you?" she asked.

"Don't you have to be licensed to do nails? I know you took classes in school because you practiced on me. I mean if you want to risk the reputation of your salon by using unqualified technicians, I'll scrub up." I replied.

"Okay fine. I'll do the manicure, but you need to be my helper and do everything I tell you to do," she declared.

"No problem boss."

"I'm sure she's still not going to tell us anything. We're just the lowly help."

"No, but she might tell another wealthy lady."

"If you and I are doing her nails and hair, who is going to play the rich, suffering housewife?" Lan asked.

"Brianna," we said in unison.

It was probably the fastest unofficial "sting operation" put together that the police department never knew about. It took us a week to get everything together. Lan had to find a day on her schedule when Ru would be out, and she could tell her cleaning staff to not come in so that the salon would be empty and our set up would not be touched. I had to also block the time on my schedule as well without arousing Adriana's ire. Lan borrowed some nail art equipment from some acquaintances in the business. Because of the nature of my profession, manicures were not very practical for me so my experiences with them were limited. I was glad that Lan was taking the lead on it. The smell of the chemicals was so toxic, I couldn't imagine how someone could do this for hours, much less days and months at a time.

We made up some flyers for a "free hair shampoo with blowout and manicure" special to pass around the neighborhood because Lan thought it would be a good promotion for her salon and she might as well get something for her troubles. When everything was set, we drove to Mrs. Ashwar's house at 11:00 p.m. on a Wednesday night to put the flyer into her mailbox. Then we waited the next day for a response. The flyer said the special was good for two days only. Lan and I didn't want the operation to happen on Saturday since it was our busiest day. I hoped and prayed Mrs. Ashwar's schedule would work for us.

Thursday morning, I stopped by Lan's house on my way to work for coffee and a pow wow. I had been leaving the house early for work several days now. Fred was getting suspicious, but I assured him everything was all right.

"How are we going to know if she's going to come?" Lan asked. "I've already gotten calls about it. People want to know how they can redeem it."

"I put a note on her flyer that it can only be redeemed by making an appointment, so she needs to call or text for an appointment time. You know, we're a classy place. No walk ins," I smirked.

"You should totally do that for your office and maybe you wouldn't be so miserable when you get a bunch of walk ins five minutes before closing," she replied.

"I wish I could girl, I wish I could. I don't think Adriana would sign off on that one."

"Who's the boss you or her?"

"Uh, I'll say it's me, but I think we both know how long I'd last if that were really the case. I enjoy the eyecare part, dealing with the pitfalls of business, not so much."

"All that schooling and training you had to go through, and this is the state of your career," she stated shaking her head.

"I never claimed to have gone into healthcare to get rich. Besides, if all I cared about was making money, I wouldn't be able to have moments like this with you," I replied.

Lan's phone buzzed announcing a new text message and she quickly grabbed it. "It's her!"

"What does she say?" I asked eagerly.

"She says she wants an appointment for Friday morning at 9:00 a.m. Woohoo! We did it!" Lan shouted, putting her hand up for a high five. I hit it and added a little happy dance.

"Of course, now comes the hardest part," I announced sadly.

"Convincing Brianna to help us?"

"Yes," I sighed dejectedly. "Let's get it over with."

I dialed up Brianna's number. She answered on the third ring.

"Hello," she answered sleepily. I forgot she didn't often get up until after 10:00 a.m.

"Brianna, my favorite sister-in-law," I gushed enthusiastically.

"I'm your only sister-in-law," she replied grumpily. Apparently, she figured that one out. "Why are you calling me so early? Don't tell me you need some more clothes."

"No, no. I'm sorry I didn't realize it was so early," I apologized. It was 8:00 a.m. "I just wanted to tell you about Friday. It's very exciting!"

"What's happening on Friday?" she asked curiously.

"Lan's doing a special day at her salon. You can get a free manicure and free haircut ..." I started, but then Lan nudged me hard in the ribs. "I mean free manicure and hair shampoo with blow out."

"Hmm. What's the catch?" she asked suspiciously.

"What makes you think there's a catch?" I replied innocently.

"Because you're calling me at 8:00 in the morning to randomly tell me this."

"I just couldn't wait to tell you is all. And we need you to come in at 9:00 a.m. exactly since it's such a popular deal and she's going to be so busy," I assured her.

"9:00?! I don't even get dressed until 9:30. I'm going to have to pass."

"No, wait. Don't hang up. Okay, here's the deal. Lan and I are helping Jaime out with a case, but we're not officially working with the police. We're setting up an undercover operation at her salon so we can get information about some burglaries in the ritzy areas of town. We need you to come in and gossip with a wealthy lady, so she'll spill the beans," I confessed.

I was too wound up to come up with some other deception. Besides, we needed Brianna to get such specific information, she had to know the truth. There were several minutes of silence. It was going on so long I thought she might have hung up.

"So, let me get this straight. You need me to come to the salon to get information from some rich lady because you think rich women will only talk to other rich ladies?" she asked bluntly.

"Well, yes." I replied losing confidence by the minute.

"Hahaha," she chortled hysterically.

"Listen," I said desperate to salvage the situation. "It's not that I think she'll talk to any rich woman, I think she'll talk to *you*. You are such a gorgeous person with a fabulous personality. You have a way of making people tell you anything. Lan and I can't do it because we're so plain."

"Speak for yourself," Lan whispered defensively.

"We need you Brianna," I pleaded while motioning Lan to hush.

"Well, why didn't you say so earlier. Of course, I can get her to tell me anything. What do you need to know?" she replied more accommodatingly.

"We believe she is a patient of a therapist down at Richmond and I-610 who is manipulating her patients to steal pricey collectibles from their husbands and pass them along to her. Trouble is, we don't have any proof. We either need to know where the items are or confirmation that this is happening."

More silence.

"I'm still going to get my free manicure and shampoo with blowout if I do this, right?" she asked finally.

"Absolutely," I said.

"I want a free color too. My roots need touching up."

Lan heard this and pursed her lips while shaking her fist at the phone.

"Deal," I agreed.

"Okay fine. I'll do it. You'll owe me one too. After all, I'm giving up my beauty sleep for you."

"Thanks Brianna. We appreciate you. See you Friday, don't be late," I said and hung up the phone.

"OMG!" exclaimed Lan. "That woman is some piece of work."

"I know, but we need her right now. Let's hope she delivers for us."

Chapter 13

L

an and I were a bundle of nerves Friday morning. I had decided to block the whole morning off from my office. I had no idea of how long this little sting operation of ours would take, but I knew I would be too distracted if I was worrying about making it back to the office to see patients. Adriana was not happy, but I agreed to double book for the afternoon and try virtual follow up exams a few nights after hours to make up for it. Technology would be the death of me sooner or later. I was heading for the door with my hair twisted up in a messy bun and flush with anticipation when Fred confronted me as I was about to leave to meet Lan at her salon.

"Something special going on at the office this morning?" he asked, standing with his arms crossed and brows raised. "You're looking more excited than usual."

"Uh, I'm actually meeting Lan this morning. She's trying out manicures in her salon and I promised I would help her set up," I replied not entirely lying.

"That's surprising. I thought she said she would never do manicures as a matter of principle."

"She's had a change of heart. Business is business you know."

I cleared my throat uncomfortably.

"That's true. You should take a lesson from her and try something new too at your office."

"Actually I am. I'm going to be doing some virtual exams for established patients a few nights a week."

"Oh. Wow. I wouldn't have expected that from you, especially with how adverse you are to technology. I remember when you even said you preferred paper exams as opposed to electronic records."

"Oh right. I guess I just didn't like having to turn my back on patients to enter data into a computer. But I can adapt, eventually. I can't help it if I'm old fashioned."

"Indeed," he replied as he picked up a doily from the kitchen counter that I had crocheted.

"That's not old fashioned, that's art," I protested. "Anyway, I've got to go. Don't want to keep her waiting. Have a good day Fred!" I chirped as I dashed out the door.

The salon looked fantastic. We brought in bouquets of fresh flowers and set up a station for coffee, pastries, even mimosas. Nothing like a little champagne to loosen lips. The place had more of a spa feeling than the usual rock n roll, artsy vibe. We even swapped out the posters of musicians and actors with edgy haircuts on the walls with pictures of fountains and the Eiffel Tower. Relaxing orchestral music played quietly in the background. Lilith Janus had nothing on us.

Thank goodness Ru was off work this morning so that he wouldn't blow our cover. I had called Brianna again last night to offer pointers on what to say and what kind of information we needed. She listened for about five minutes and then said she would get the information her own way.

It was going to be a crazy day, but all worth it, if it worked out. The last time I felt this type of exhilaration was the first time I had to do an entire eye exam myself during clinical rotations in optometry school. Only this time, if I screwed up, no one would lose an eye or two.

"Are you ready?" I asked Lan as I finished setting up the manicure station and put my apron on.

"I think so. How about you? You're going to be pretending to not know English. It's going to be hard for you to not speak," she laughed.

"Yes, and even harder putting our fate in Brianna's hands," I lamented.

The clock hands pointed to five minutes past 9:00 a.m. Our hope was diminishing. Then the door opened, and Mrs. Ashwar came in. She was heavier set than the internet pictures of her showed. They were apparently older pictures. She looked sullen and unsure if she wanted to stay. Lan and I quickly welcomed her in before she had a chance to leave.

"Welcome! Welcome! Mrs. Ashwar?" Lan gushed with a slight Vietnamese accent.

I smiled and bowed repeatedly. I gestured to come in and take a seat in the salon chair.

"Yes, I'm Mrs. Ashwar," she responded. She looked around and decided it was safe to stay. "Am I the only one here?" she asked, taking a seat in the chair.

"Yes, for now. We are only taking clients in small groups to offer you a beautiful and peaceful experience," Lan explained. "My name is Lan. May I offer you some refreshment?" she asked and then barked some orders to me in Vietnamese.

I nodded profusely and scurried over to get a fluted glass of mimosa and a pastry. I brought it to Mrs. Ashwar on a

silver-plated tray and set it down on a little table next to
Mrs. Ashwar's chair. I bowed again and waited to see what
she would do. She thanked me and picked up the drink and
sniffed at it before taking a drink.

"Thi-na is new. I am training her today. She doesn't
speak much English," Lan informed her. "What color
would you like for today? We have lots of beautiful colors.
Makes your hands and feet look special and wealthy. It will
make your husband smile."

Lan was doing a bang-up job. Maybe I should try and
get her to sell glasses for me. Mrs. Ashwar picked a
shimmery purple and gold color. I put the little bottles on
the manicure table and then led her to the hair washing
station and gestured that she should sit down and lean back
to get her hair washed. She complied reluctantly. Then I
gestured if I could take her shoes off.

"You want to take my shoes?" she asked surprised. I
nodded, smiling coyly the whole time.

"She wants to help you feel comfortable. We have these
disposable slippers for you to wear that you can take home
with you," Lan explained. "Since you are our first customer
today, we will also give you a free pedicure too."

"Oh, okay," she acquiesced. It's hard to turn down free
stuff.

It was a clever move by Lan. A pedicure would keep her
in the salon longer. Taking away her shoes was another way
of making sure she didn't get up and escape before we had
what we needed. I quickly removed her shoes and put the
slippers on. I put a towel around her shoulders and leaned
her head back. I turned on the water faucet to start rinsing
her hair in the sink. However, I was not familiar with the
faucet, so I turned it on full blast. The force of the water
gushing out sent a tidal wave of water over the sink. I

yelped in panic as water splashed everywhere. Lan ran over to rescue me. She yelled at me in Vietnamese which roughly translated to, "Heavens woman! You're not trying to wash a dog. Get it together."

After the wash, we escorted Mrs. Ashwar to the salon chairs to dry and style her hair. At least I could work the pump on the chair to make her rise. It was a bit different using a manual pump since my office uses an automatic one, but potato, potato. I got out of Lan's way so she could style Mrs. Ashwar's hair. Watching her work, I was amazed at how confidently and skillfully she used a brush and hair dryer. She was very good at what she did.

I went to get Mrs. Ashwar another pastry and glanced at the clock. It was already 9:15 and no sign of Brianna. I hope she wasn't going to let us down. Lan and I exchanged worried looks, so we decided we might have to go to plan B and try to get Mrs. Ashwar to confide in us.

"So, a beautiful lady like you, you must be married," Lan inquired cheerily.

"Yes, I'm married," Mrs. Ashwar replied sipping her mimosa.

"Oh yes, I see your beautiful ring. Your husband must love you a lot. Have you been married for a long time? My husband and I been married for 3 years, but we still feel like newlyweds you know what I mean?" she chuckled winking and smiling.

"I've been married for ten years. It feels like ten years," she replied dryly.

Lan burst out laughing. I chuckled as well.

"That's a good one," she chortled. "I understand that. Some men don't know how to be married. Makes you feel crazy like you have to go get therapy, you know what I mean?"

157

"No, what do you mean by that?" she asked suspiciously.

"Uh nothing Ma'am. Just talking. Would you like some more mimosa to drink?" Lan asked trying to play it cool.

"Yes, I'll have another drink," she said drinking down what was left in her glass.

I quickly came over and took her empty glass and replaced it with a full one. Lan finished her hair. It looked fabulous and she complimented Lan on it. The great hair and second mimosa were starting to relax her. We moved her to the manicure station.

We started with her pedicure so we could whisper together on what the backup plan would be. It was determined that we didn't have much chance to get information on what Lilith Janus might have told her, but if we could at least establish that she was a patient of Ms. Janus and link that with the timing of her husband's police burglary filing, that might be something. We were running out of time. If we finished her manicure before Brianna came, it would all have been for naught. The room was silent except for the light music. The feeling was awkward. Suddenly the door swung open and in walked Brianna decked out in designer everything including some giant high-end sunglasses with gold and cream-colored frames and grey tinted lenses that seemed to swallow half her face. I had gifted those to her for her birthday. They were the only gift she ever liked from me.

"Hello ladies, I'm here for my appointment," she announced strutting in on her stilettos and carrying her handbag on her arm.

"Oh Mrs. Trí. So good of you to come," Lan exclaimed with a hint of sarcasm. "Please come and have a seat here." Lan sat her in the chair next to Mrs. Ashwar. "I'll be with you soon. Can we get you some refreshments?"

"I'll have what she's having," Brianna replied nonchalantly as she placed her very expensive purse down on the table in front of Mrs. Ashwar where it could be seen. As she seated herself down, she made a show of removing her sunglasses and adjusting the rings on her fingers. Then she turned to Mrs. Ashwar and introduced herself.

"Hello. I'm Brianna Trí. How are they treating you here?"

"Hello. I'm Ruchi Ashwar. It's been very pleasant here," Mrs. Ashwar replied.

Sounds like our attempts at a relaxing spa treatment was working. I brought Brianna a mimosa, a pastry and a magazine and went back to helping Lan with Mrs. Ashwar. I kept my head down and took Mrs. Ashwar's nails out of the soaking liquid and was toweling them off so I wouldn't have to look at Brianna. Brianna took a big sip of her mimosa and smacked her lips.

"Mmm, just what I needed after a tough morning shopping. I needed a little retail therapy," she crowed.

Everyone smiled politely to Brianna, but no one said anything.

"I like the colors you picked," Brianna said to Mrs. Ashwar. "It reminds me of the dress I wore when my husband Vu proposed to me."

"Oh really?" Mrs. Ashwar replied politely.

"Yes, that was a beautiful night. When my Vu finally made enough money to ask me to make him the happiest man on Earth," she recounted.

I was twisting the towel in my hands and grinding my teeth. It was also the night the rest of us wondered, why her? He could have done so much better.

159

"That's nice," Mrs. Ashwar smiled, no doubt feeling mellow from her mimosas.

"Yes, it was wonderful. Little did I know what I was in for," her tone changing from wistful to bitter. "After we were married, he was out every night drinking and gambling," she scowled. "I told him, you keep this up and you won't have enough money to keep me. But did he listen? No. Finally, I had to find a way to get his attention. At least that's what my therapist told me to do."

"Oh yeah?" Mrs. Ashwar replied, her ears perking up.

"Yeah, she said I should take something precious to him and tuck it away somewhere safe where he couldn't find it. Then when he's wallowing in misery because he can't find it, poof. I should swoop in and remind him that he didn't need it to make him happy because that's what I was for. When I heard that, I thought to myself, that's the most ridiculous thing I ever heard. But then I figured what the hell. For the amount of money that I'm paying that therapist, maybe it's worth a shot. So, I took his lucky Rolex watch and 24k gold cufflinks. He was hysterical when he couldn't find it," she whispered as if she was confiding in Mrs. Ashwar.

"And did it work?" Mrs. Ashwar asked eagerly. She was completely engrossed in Brianna's story.

"It did," Brianna said. "It was a good plan. That Lilith Janus is a genius."

"Is that your therapist?" Mrs. Ashwar asked with obvious surprise.

"It is. Her office is over on Richmond and I-610. Trouble is, she double crossed me," Brianna declared angrily.

"What do you mean?" Mrs. Ashwar asked anxiously.

"I asked that uptight secretary of hers to get my stuff back and she said I couldn't have it back because part of the plan was that Janus should hold onto it indefinitely. But between you and me, I'm sure she sold it. I slipped that secretary some money to tell me."

"What?!" Mrs. Ashwar exclaimed in shock and practically spitting out her mimosa.

"That's right. That manipulating therapist did a number on me. She convinces me to hand over my husband's very precious and very expensive things, and then sells them right under my nose. I guess she figured I'd be so happy that my marriage was saved that I'd forget about them or something."

Mrs. Ashwar's face blanched and then flushed with color. She was visibly shaken. Lan had just finished her manicure when she tried to get up.

"Is something wrong honey?" Brianna asked innocently.

"No, I just have to go," she exclaimed and started reaching for her purse.

"Wet, wet," I said and motioned to her fingers and toes.

"Well, if you're feeling upset for me, don't worry honey I'm going to get the good doctor back," Brianna confided confidently.

"What do you mean?" Mrs. Ashwar asked sitting back down.

"You see my Vu is a lawyer, a very successful lawyer. When I told him what happened, he was furious. We're going to sue her for malpractice. She abused her position and took advantage of me in a vulnerable state. Not to mention theft. He says we'd have a stronger case if we could find someone else that she might have done this to as well. The problem is, I don't know anyone else who has gone to see her. I don't think she'd give us a list of her patients. HIPAA violation or something," Brianna said sipping her mimosa calmly.

Mrs. Ashwar was silent. We all held our breath. It seemed like she was weighing whether to say something or not. She glanced at me and Lan, so I put my head down and started cleaning up the manicure tools and supplies.

Lan walked over to the far end of the salon and was tidying up things to give Mrs. Ashwar space to confide in Brianna. Brianna was flipping through her magazine and looking every bit the spoiled housewife, so Mrs. Ashwar finally leaned over towards her.

"I think I can help you," she whispered.

"You can?" Brianna asked innocently.

"Yes, I am a patient of Lilith Janus too. I can join your case."

"Why my prayers are answered. Thank you, Mrs. Ashwar. I'm so glad to have met you. Tell you what, here's my name and phone number. You call me soon okay, and we'll get some justice," Brianna told her while handing her one of Vu's business cards with her name and number written on the back.

I shot a look at Lan and nodded to signal that we got what we needed. She walked back over to Mrs. Ashwar smiling widely.

"Thank you for coming today. We hope to see you again soon," Lan cooed.

Mrs. Ashwar started to put her shoes on. That's when Brianna saw her pedicure and started to pitch a fit.

"She got a pedicure too! How come you only offered me a manicure?" she shrieked.

I was so startled I dropped my nail clippers on the floor and when I bent down to pick it up, I lost my footing and lunged forward.

"Oh no!" I cried and tried to grab something to catch myself. Instead, I ended up knocking a tray over and spilling bowls of liquid, towels and nail polish that landed on me before finishing with a great clatter on the floor.

Brianna started cackling, so Lan rushed Mrs. Ashwar out the door before anything else could go wrong. I don't know if I would ever be able to live down the humiliation, but I took comfort in the fact that our scheme had worked. For all her bad qualities, I had to admit that Brianna came through for us.

I showed up to work a bit disheveled, but in relatively good spirits. Adriana looked at me with her silent, disapproving, matriarchal expression.

"So, you took the morning off to get a manicure? You reek of acetone. And why is there paint in your hair?" she asked, her expression unchanged.

"Uh well, I had an accident this morning with some nail polish. I'll go fix my hair and soak my hands in some peroxide. At least that smells a bit more sanitary," I replied quietly to avoid any more confrontation. I trudged into my office to put away my purse and slipped on my white clinic jacket.

"What kind of accident could you have by just putting nail polish on?" she called to me from the front desk.

"It's a long story, but let's just say I now have new sympathy for patients that accidentally injure themselves putting make-up on their eyes."

Chapter 14

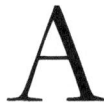

s I sat in my office sipping my morning tea pensively, I shared my thoughts aloud, "A famous person once said, 'there are people who have money and people who are rich'."

Although I enjoyed the smell of coffee, I didn't drink it. It made me too jittery, and I was anxious enough at times.

"Who said that?" asked Adriana. "Confucious? Buddha? The Dalai lama?"

"Coco Chanel," I replied with gravitas.

"And then there are people who need to pay their bills and would like a little money left over to have a life," Adriana retorted as she rolled her eyes. "Only people with a lot of money would go around saying nonsense like that. If you're telling me this to make up for blocking the morning schedule the other day, it's not going to work. We're still short of making our monthly goal and frankly I'm getting pretty tired of it."

"I know," I replied ruefully. "I'm sorry about that. I know how hard you work to keep this place afloat, but it was necessary."

"Hanging out with your best friend, doing some rich lady's nails to get information is not what I consider that important as far as our business goes," she scolded. "How did it turn out anyway? Is that Lilith Janus going to jail?"

I didn't intend to let Adriana know what we were up to, but I had run out of Lan's salon so quickly to get to work that Brianna felt the need to call the office and let everyone know what had transpired.

"It turned out great. Not only was Brianna good at playing the rich, injured housewife and manipulating Lilith Janus's victim to turn on her, but she was also responsible enough to connect Mrs. Ashwar to Jaime who took her statement down. From there he had evidence to issue a warrant and searched Lilith Janus's home and office. They found the stolen items in her office."

"Where in the world did she keep stuff in her office? In that area of town, rent is crazy expensive. It can't be a very big place."

"There were three, large, custom-built safes hidden behind some nature paintings in her office," I replied.

"How did they know to look there?"

"I suggested they look there. When I was in her office, I noticed these paintings. The paintings were so large and the images so striking that you wouldn't normally pay much attention to the frames. But since I was scoping the place out during my undercover visit, I noticed the darkness and shadows on the wall from where they protruded away from it. I knew it couldn't be just a perception thing, but that there was three-dimensional depth behind the paintings. A good place to hide a safe."

"Of course. I should have known you'd figure it out Dr. Trí. Had she sold any of the items?"

"Not any of the items that had an open police report. Only items that were never reported or whose files had been closed as non-recoverable because the statute of limitation had run out."

"Did you know for sure that she had the stolen items and had planned to sell them before your little 'sting operation' at Lan's salon?"

"Not entirely," I admitted. "We just did a little psychological manipulating of our own on Mrs. Ashwar to make her think Janus sold off her husband's prized Atari collection. Lilith Janus had promised her no harm would come to it. Of course, there is something I can't quite figure out."

"What's that?"

"She is an attractive woman with great credentials and good at her job. It puzzles me why she would even want to resort to stealing, and in this way. I mean her exam fees alone feels like robbery but at least they're legal and would set her up well. I wonder if she had a partner, or someone manipulated her into this nefarious activity."

"Or maybe she's just greedy. For some people, too much is never enough," Adriana declared not interested in delving into the criminal mind. "Of course, if we don't get more high paying patients, we may have to resort to something like that."

"Yeah right," I laughed but Adriana didn't. "You are kidding right?"

Adriana gave me a cryptic look as she left to go to her desk. The light went on for the internal number on my office phone. A signal that my next patient was ready.

"Good morning Mr. Smith. How are you doing today?" I asked the first patient as I sat down on my doctor's stool and pulled up his chart on the computer.

"Good morning, Dr. Trí," he replied. "I could be better. I had my full exam a few months ago, but in the last week my eyes have been red, itchy, and watery. They feel swollen."

I typed in the symptoms he had described into his chart. Then I looked at him. Indeed, the clear membrane on top of the whites of his eyes were quite swollen and weepy looking. In addition, the whites of his eyes were pink all over. Itchy, watery, swollen conjunctival membranes usually meant one thing, allergy.

"Mr. Smith do you normally have allergies? For example, do your eyes get itchy and watery to things in the environment like dust, grass, or pollen?"

"Not really. Maybe if the pollen count is high when I'm mowing the lawn my eyes may water and my nose may run, but I'll usually wear a mask if I'm going to be doing anything like that. And anyway, I haven't been outside much lately."

"I see. Have you changed your laundry detergent lately, or started using new soap?" I continued in my questioning.

"No, that's all the same."

"Have you gotten a new pet or touched someone else's pet recently?"

"No, not that either."

"Have you been cleaning out your house where there was a lot of dust or mold?"

"No. I don't remember doing anything like that."

"Do you remember rubbing your eyes recently?"

"Not really," he replied growing impatient. "I've already told you I haven't changed anything in my life, so you'll have to figure something else out doctor."

I could see I needed to take a different approach to get some answers. Mr. Smith was usually so pleasant, but today something must be bothering him. It would be easy enough to prescribe eyedrop medication to treat the current condition. However, without knowing the source of the condition, there would continue to be flare ups and treatment could go on indefinitely.

To calm him, I decided to move on to the objective testing to confirm the diagnosis and continue the questioning later. His vision was close to normal with his glasses on. His eye movements were intact although he noted his eyes felt uncomfortable when he moved them around, like "a pressure". Looking with my slit lamp, I observed his anterior eye structures and found them all normal. I instilled some eye dye to observe if he had any superficial abrasions or dry patches that may be causing the irritation and swelling and found nothing of note. His outer eyelids were also swollen, likely from the profuse tearing. Due to this swelling, I had difficulty checking under his eyelids. He winced and complained of discomfort. There were large, clear, cyst like bumps on the inside of his lower and upper eyelids. A definite indication of allergy.

"Mr. Smith, you are definitely having an allergic reaction to something. We can treat it with some eyedrop medication, but I want you to think very carefully about what you have been doing lately as well as the places you have been to in the last week. Did you go somewhere you normally don't?"

He sighed, but then was quiet thinking and replaying the events of the week in his mind.

"Gosh, it has been such a stressful week," he acknowledged. "My wife just got diagnosed with early-stage breast cancer."

"Oh, I'm so sorry."

"Thank you. I think we caught it early but there has been lots of doctors' visits."

"I can imagine."

"Also, my daughter is getting a divorce, so I have been watching her kids for her. Come to think of it, I did take them to a place that gives hayrides. I suppose there was a lot of hay dust in the air."

"And did you wipe your eyes with your hands or with your shirt at all?"

"It's hard to remember, but it's possible that I did. Do you think you it could be the hay?"

"I think that's a strong possibility or the dust or whatever was with the hay."

"Does that mean I'm allergic to hay and I should avoid it?"

"I can't say for sure, but it helps to be aware that you might be. We want to treat your symptoms but also eliminate the source, if possible," I counseled him as I entered the prescription into the computer and hit print. "I suppose if you really wanted to know you could do a provocative test," I added jocosely.

"What do you mean?" he asked. "What is a provocative test?"

"It's when you want to know if something will cause an adverse or hypersensitive response, such as an allergic reaction, you expose yourself to it. For example, when this allergic reaction that you've had is resolved, you could visit the hay bales again and see what happens. But please be careful, it can be hazardous to your health running headlong into danger just to get a reaction."

I printed out a prescription for the eyedrop medication and handed it to Mr. Smith.

"Take this medication as I have instructed and come back in a few days so we can follow up with you to make sure it's all better."

"Okay Dr. Trí," he agreed. "I hope it works. I called my family doctor about it, and he suggested I use some over-the-counter allergy drops like, Clear Up Your Eyes. It hasn't helped."

"Not for something like this. You are having such a severe allergic reaction that you need medication. You did right to come see me," I assured him.

"Thank you and sorry about being short with you earlier," he apologized as I walked him out to the front desk.

"I understand. Our emotions get away from us when life is stressful. Have a great day," I smiled.

It was nice to have a pleasant patient periodically. The constant stream of people taking out their "bad day" on you is not good for your mental health. I'm only human after all.

Chapter 15

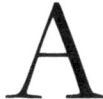driana walked into my office and declared, "Bad news doc."

"Only bad news? What about, 'I have good news and bad news which do you want first'?"

"Okay, I have bad news and worse news which do you want first?" she replied sarcastically.

"Okay give me the bad news first."

"I got a letter from our management. They are raising our rent to twice as much as it was."

"What!" I shouted in disbelief. "They can't do that! Can they?"

"I'm not a lawyer but seems to me if it's their building they can do as they please."

"Our lease is up this year. They know that, so they're putting the squeeze on us. I'll have to ask my brother about it. I'm afraid to ask but what's the worse news?"

"John has given his two-week notice," she stated sadly.

"What!" I shouted again incredulously. "Why? He seemed so happy here with us."

"Apparently sometimes happiness is not enough, or maybe it comes in different forms for different people," she replied cryptically.

"I looked at her face and thought about her words. It's money, isn't it? Is he going to Dr. Moore's office?"

"I'm afraid so. Wow Dr. Trí, you do have great powers of deductive reasoning."

"It doesn't take a great detective to see that we're scraping along while they're making money hand over fist over there. Has he tried to recruit you again too?"

"He has."

"What's keeping you here? The challenge? The excitement of financial uncertainty," I asked woefully.

"Funny," she replied. "I'd be lying if I said I hadn't thought about it before. The extra money would be good, but it's a meat market over there. Every day they are rushing patients through and constantly looking to see if they've met their goals for bonuses."

"But you're always keeping track to see if we've met our financial goals for the month here."

"Yes, but at least it's to benefit the entire office. There, it's set up more so that people are competing with each other instead of like a team. The office politics are brutal. Sure, they're all smiling to your face, but people are constantly stabbing each other in the back to get ahead. If I had wanted that type of stress, I would go work at Allmart."

"Hellooo. Knock, knock," came a voice outside the office. "I hope you don't mind my coming back here instead of waiting in the optical dispensary. Your receptionist wasn't at the desk, and I wanted to make sure you knew I was here."

It was Ally Gallagher, the contact lens and eyedrops sales representative for Genericeye Corporation. Genericeye

Corporation was one of the big companies in the eye business. They made contact lenses, contact lens cleaners, dry eye moisturizing drops, eye allergy medication, etc. Her appointment was supposed to be at lunch time, but she was early.

"Ally, so good to see you," I said politely standing up to greet her. "You look fabulous. I love those blue high heeled shoes you're wearing. What is that suede?"

"Thank you. They are leather *and* suede, for comfort *and* style," she grinned. "They cost a bundle, but I love them so much it was worth it."

"Life's too short, right? You're early. I thought we were doing a lunch meeting?"

"And how long have you been standing there?" Adriana asked suspiciously.

"Oh well, I just came in a minute ago and I do have a lunch order for some barbecue to be delivered to the office. I was so excited to come tell you about our new products that I didn't think you would mind if I came in a little early."

"We do mind. That's what appointments are for, so we're not tied up with patients," Adriana stated flatly. She was none too pleased with the intrusion.

"Of course, but it doesn't look like there are any patients at the moment," she replied smiling.

"Yes, well I'm looking forward to hearing about your new product. Let me check the schedule to make sure there aren't any imminent patients," I interjected.

"Actually, I took the liberty to peek at your schedule out there and it seems that your next patient has rescheduled and there wasn't an appointment after that, so you should be free," she said with her savvy, salesperson smile.

"Okay, I guess I'm available then. Won't you have a seat," I offered motioning to a chair opposite to me.

"I'll leave you to it. I need to talk with Dora about leaving the schedule up when she's away from her station," Adriana muttered as she excused herself and left.

"So efficient and hardworking that Adriana, isn't she?" Ally commented after Adriana was out of the office. "I hope you're paying her well. It's so hard to find good help these days."

"Yes, it is. I'm very lucky she's happy here. We're a good team. Now what have you got for me?" I asked, eager to change the subject.

"It's still pending FDA approval, but we are in the final phase of clinical trials for a new type of eyelash gel that will grow your eyelashes fuller!" she exclaimed excitedly while taking out a stack of paperwork.

"Is it supposed to be for hypotrichosis which results in little to no hair growth on the head? This of course would include the eyelashes."

"Yes, that's what it's officially for. However, just like that other brand that started out as medication for something else, it can also be used for cosmetic purposes as long as you get evaluated for it from your eye doctor, of course. It's called Plaintoful eyelash gel. Although if you use a separate brush, I'm sure you could use it on your eyebrows too," she winked and handed me several brochures and information sheets.

"I see what you did there," I chuckled at the name. "So, you will be competing with the other eyelash growing product?" I asked, glancing at the charts and diagrams trying to make sense of it.

"Yes, but we're on a whole other level than them. Our growth mechanism is different from theirs and far superior in my opinion. It's thought that their formulation extends the part of the growth phase of the eyelash to grow longer.

It's not for sure, but whatever chemicals they are using to do this is probably what's causing the added side effects of pigmentation and irritation at the base of the eyelashes. Ours is more holistic in that it uses a blend of nutritional vitamins and growth hormones that encourage more eyelashes to grow at the same time instead of a normal staggered growth pattern giving you thicker, fuller looking lashes."

"Hmm, that's interesting," I replied reading through the paperwork, but not really getting any hard evidence, just a lot of fantastical sales pitches and promises. "Do you have any studies that I could look at?"

"The company told me that the information is proprietary. But they are doing legitimate studies. I'm in one of the trials too."

"You are?" I asked surprised.

"Sure am. See my lashes," she said blinking her eyes alluringly. "I'm not even wearing any mascara."

"Wow," I exclaimed looking at the dense growth of eyelashes on her eyes. "Do you have a before picture by chance?"

"Yes, let me look on my phone. I usually am wearing false eyelashes or mascara before I started participating in the study, so I need to find a picture where I'm just at home," she confessed as she scrolled through the pictures on her smartphone. "Ah, here we go. Please excuse the way I'm dressed. I was taking my dog on a walk."

I looked at the picture and sure enough, there she was smiling makeup free and with just a thin line of sparse eyelashes. It was a real contrast compared to her normal appearance which was all made up from head to toe. She often came in well dressed, with her hair done in a nice blow out and lots of make-up. I figured it was part of a salesperson's uniform. Maybe that's why I didn't sell many high-end frames and "premium" contact lenses. My usual look encompassed my hair tied into a simple ponytail and a swipe of neutral colored lipstick to keep my lips from chapping. No fuss, no muss was my mantra.

"Excuse me, may I?" Ally asked as she pointed to a tissue box on my desk.

"Sure, help yourself."

"Thank you," she replied gratefully as she took a tissue and dabbed her eyes. "It's a good thing that I don't have to wear any mascara the way my eyes have been running lately."

"Oh, do you have allergies?" I asked.

"I have some seasonal allergies, but I take allergy pills for those when needed. Ironically, my eyes are usually very dry. No this started a few months after I started in the clinical trials. I asked the researchers about it. They said a few other subjects were getting this side effect too. They think the gel is also stimulating the tear glands to work more as well. They figured it was a bonus feature to offer more moisture to the eyes. They're thinking of marketing it as a dry eye treatment too."

"Goodness, the one miracle drug to cure all ocular ails. Does it fix presbyopia too? Then you would have gold on your hands."

"I wish," she laughed. "Then I would be able to retire. Full disclosure, I just bought stock in the company."

"You really have faith in this product, don't you?"

"I sure do." She was grinning from ear to ear.

"Pardon me if I'm being too nosey, but is there something more?" I inquired.

"No," she said coyly, but unable to stop smiling. I gave her a raised eyebrow and penetrating stare. "Okay, but if I tell you, it's just between you and me."

"Of course," I agreed.

"I'm dating one of the researchers at Genericeye Corporation. In fact, he's the head researcher for the Plaintoful eyelash gel."

"Do tell," I urged very interested.

"His name is Dr. Tristan Brone. He has a Ph.D. in biochemistry, and he's been at Genericeye Corporation for a few years. However, this is the first project that he's overseen. He says if it passes FDA approval, it could be a game changer for the company and the field. He'll be rich and ready to propose too!"

"Wow, that's incredible and very exciting for the both of you. Congratulations. But." I hesitated.

"What is it?" she asked concerned that anything would destroy all her hopes and dreams.

"Do you think your enthusiasm for the efficacy of this drug is colored by your relationship to Dr. Brone? I mean, these glossy brochures are nice to look at, but they're not really telling me anything substantial about the product. Do you have any peer reviewed articles on the studies themselves?"

"No. They aren't releasing those. It's proprietary information," she insisted. "Besides, I've met his boss who is vice president of the company, Mr. Cooper. He is a stickler for details, and he says he wouldn't release anything that wasn't totally safe."

I must have had a skeptical expression because she softened her tone.

"I understand your concern. What do you want to know about it?"

"First of all, what exactly is in it?"

"That's proprietary."

"Well then, how was it tested? Were there control groups? Was it a double-blind study? Were the results statistically significant? Were there any side effects or negative results? What are the long-term effects?" I persisted.

"Whoa, slow down," she said overwhelmed by my line of questioning. "You are one curious doctor. I, for sure, do not have answers for all those questions. If you like, I can try and get them from Tristan. Why don't you give me a question I can answer."

"Fair enough. Will the company be releasing a standard application procedure for patients and monitoring schedule for doctors so that we can make sure patients are using it safely? I presume it will be by prescription."

"Yes. Especially since it is so new. Just between you and me, I overheard that if the product does well, in a couple of years it will be released as an over-the-counter product."

"What?" I exclaimed, alarmed. "This type of thing has to be monitored. If it's over-the-counter, patients will never come in to make sure nothing goes wrong. Who knows what it could be doing to them?"

"I agree with you. I think it's important to be careful and to support our doctors as partners in eyecare and with eyecare products, but money talks you know."

"I do, unfortunately."

"Besides, it's supposed to be a natural product. How much harm could it do?"

"Said the makers of cigarettes before people started dying from cancer due to secondhand smoke," I answered sarcastically. "But pay no attention to me. I'm a skeptic until I know all the facts. Do you have a sample?"

"I understand. That's why I like talking with you. I know if I can convince you of our product's worth, you'll be able to convince your patients. I've watched you with them. You spend more time explaining things to them to make sure they understand what's going on with their eyes and why they need the treatment you prescribe."

"Thank you, Ally. That's kind of you to say. Be sure to tell Adriana that on your way out so she won't be so upset with me when I'm running late on the schedule."

"Ha-ha, she does like to crack the whip, doesn't she?"

"Yes, and thank goodness for it, or I would have gone out of business long ago."

"I am not really supposed to give too many of these out, but I want to give you one," she said and rummaged through her purse.

It was so full that she had to take items out and place them on my desk to find what she was looking for. One of the items was a small bottle of artificial tears for moisturizing the eyes. The exterior was coated with makeup.

"Ally, you must take better care of your eyedrop bottles. What if this makeup got into your eyes or caused an infection?" I chastised.

"Goodness, it does look a mess doesn't it. I keep it in my purse. My eyes used to be so dry that I was always putting a drop in it," she replied embarrassed. "It looks much worse on the outside. The inside dropper is clean." She unscrewed the top of the bottle. There was a small bit of mascara around the collar of the dropper. She frowned. "I guess you were right Dr. Trí. I was probably getting makeup in my eyes."

"Don't worry about it, Ally. Now you know," I reassured her.

She continued to look for something when finally, she found it.

"Eureka!" she exclaimed and handed me a small, long, cylindrical, vial that looked like a tube of mascara. "Use it wisely."

I turned it over in my hands. The color of the container was chartreuse green with the word Plaintoful imprinted on it in big black lettering. An eye-catching choice. When you unscrewed it and pulled it open, there was long bristly brush (similar to a spoolie mascara brush) attached to the cap. The gel was stored in the bottom of the longer tube. It was clear and thick and smelled earthy.

"Interesting delivery system. Would you put it on like you would put on mascara?"

"Almost. Except you don't put any on the length and tips of the lashes. You just wiggle it at the lash base to stimulate the cells there. It also delivers the gel nearer the waterline of the lid instead of smearing it on the external eyelid. This will produce less skin irritation since it's spread on less of the eyelid."

"I see," I replied fascinated. "I presume it's hypoallergenic and doesn't contain much preservative agents that would irritate the eye since putting it there would cause it to melt into the eyes. What is the shelf life of one bottle?"

"Good question. I believe once you open it, you need to use it every day until it's all gone. And once you stop using it, the effects will go away when the eyelashes fall out naturally."

"So, once you start, you need to keep using it indefinitely to keep up the effects," I restated. "That's a genius product for Genericeye Corporation. I'm sure they have spent millions of dollars developing this. But of course, there's the physical safety aspect we need to think about.

For example, just like with mascara, some people may accidently scratch their corneas with this brush. The bristles are placed all around the tip of the handle unlike the other brand whose brush is more like a flat paint brush."

"Genericeye Corporation has thought about that too," she replied as she returned everything she took out of her purse, back into it. "The second part of my new product presentation is this new contact lens, the Plaintoful contact lens."

She pulled out more brochures and some sample flat packages with contact lenses sealed in them.

"Are you saying these are contact lenses to be worn with the gel?" I asked a little confused.

"Yes. You put the contact lens on first to protect the eye and then you apply the Plaintoful gel. That way, you have a barrier in case you accidentally bump the brush against the eye. The contact lens parameters are similar to our current contact lenses so they can be available right away."

"Then what's new about them?"

"They come with or without power and the outer layer has a more durable coating to stand up to the brush bristles of the Plaintoful gel. That way anyone, whether they have a spectacle prescription or not, can wear the contact lenses after they've applied the gel if they like because they come in clear or colors."

I must have looked a little horrified with this application scenario because Ally's demeanor changed from cheery salesperson to serious company advocate.

"Let me get this straight. In order to use the product, people who don't need to wear any correction, will also need to wear contact lenses to apply it?"

"It's for their safety," she stated defensively. "I understand what you're saying Dr. Trí. It's an extra step and procedure for people to go through, but you'd be surprised what people will do for beauty. Besides, I doubt if they would really even need to wear the contacts. If you feel the bristles on the brush, they're actually very soft. The company has taken great pains to make everything safe for the consumer."

I felt the bristles and they were softer than a typical mascara brush, but they were still stiff enough to potentially cause a corneal abrasion. I looked at the contact lenses through the packaging and they appeared to be very similar to their regular soft contact lenses.

"So then are the Plaintoful contact lenses only recommended for people who are using the Plaintoful eyelash gel?"

"That's what we recommend, although there isn't a reason why anyone who wants them couldn't wear them. It will be good for people and you doctors because it will promote getting an eye exam. Especially since you have to be fitted for contact lenses."

"That's assuming people will follow the rules. I anticipate there will be a black market for this if it catches on. How is Genericeye Corporation going to regulate the distribution?"

"Are you sure you don't have a law degree Dr. Tri? You sure think about so many things. I haven't been told yet about that aspect, but I'm sure they will only supply them to doctors' offices and pharmacies. Between you and me, I'm sure once it becomes part of the cultural landscape and people are used to it, they can probably use the Plaintoful eyelash gel without the contacts. People wear mascara now, and there's no big medical warning labels and training that they need to go through. I'm sure you've seen many mascara brush eye injuries."

"My fair share. You are also right on that count. Even so, it sure sounds a lot like double dipping to me," I rebuked.

I was amazed at the creative depths that some companies go to for profits. Not only will they make money from selling the Plaintoful eyelash gel, but they'll also make money from selling the accompanying contact lenses to people who wouldn't need it otherwise. A masterclass in capitalism.

"Don't let it bother you Dr. Trí. You doctors will do the exams and be able to make money from it."

"Yes, money can be good. We all must make a living," I agreed with her. "But I got into optometry to also help people. This just seems like we're trying to convince people that they need something that they don't, and in the process, potentially be creating additional risk."

"You can't think of it that way. We're just giving people what they want. Instead, think of how you would be helping people."

"How do you figure?"

"People spend millions of dollars on eye make-up like mascara and eyeliner or false eyelashes. Not to mention eyelash curlers to accentuate their looks and feel better about themselves, right?"

"Yes, I can't argue with that."

"And as you say, in the process of applying these things they potentially can injure themselves on top of the money they've spent buying these items. With our product, they will be able to achieve similar enhancements to their looks without the same dangers. Not to mention the money they will save on not having to buy makeup, false eyelashes, curlers, etc. We're giving them a feasible and more natural alternative. I'd say that's helping people."

"You make a good point, but I would be careful about taking on the beauty industry. I imagine tangling with big corporations is risky business."

"Don't worry about me Dr. Trí. That's for the people in charge to deal with. I'm just a single salesperson. I mean how much of a danger could I be, right?"

"Don't sell yourself short Ally. You are good at promoting products, but you do seem to care about people too. My office is small compared to others, but you come see me and spend time with me just as much as the bigger offices out there. I appreciate that."

"Thanks Dr. Trí. I do my best," she beamed with pride. "Listen Dr. Trí. Would you mind if I didn't stay for lunch? I want to finish up my visits as soon as possible today."

"That's fine. Do you have a hot date to get to?" I teased.

"I wish. I'm trying to get my accounts in order so I can get ready for the Eyesight Expo Convention in San Diego. I just have one more office to visit."

"Which office?" I asked being nosey.

"The Southeast Texas Lasik Center. I'm meeting with Dr. Lassiere. Between you and me, the sooner I get done with his office the better."

"Why is that?"

"There was an incident some time ago that I don't want to get into, but he's been vile to me ever since."

"I'm sorry to hear that. I've never met or interacted with him before, but I've heard patients talk about him. It has been mixed reviews. People either love him or hate him. Not too much in between, curiously."

"I can believe that. He presents himself as professional and amiable, but he has quite the temper."

"The big names usually do. Couldn't you see one of the other doctors? There are several optometrists and ophthalmologists there. How about one of them?"

"He's the one in charge of our account. It's okay. I'm a professional. I'll deal with it."

"Indeed, you are. Let's change the subject to something more pleasant, the Eyesight Expo. Is it time for that already?"

"Yes, will you be going this year?"

"I would love to go. It's usually a good way for me to get all my continuing education hours done for the year and I usually run into old classmates and colleagues there. But I don't know if I should take time off the schedule for it. It's half the week. I think Adriana would have my head if I took so much time off right now."

"Oh, but you should go. We will be unveiling the Plaintoful eyelash gel and contact lenses there. There will be a big booth with lots of free items (freebies) and even a dinner, although that's on an invite only basis," she said trailing off on those last words before renewing her enthusiasm. "They're also only going to allow a few offices per area to be able to prescribe it initially. That will make it more desirable you know. Supply and demand."

"I would expect nothing less. How will they decide which office it goes to?"

"They will leave it up to your local representative," she said smiling and batting her eyes. "And as one of my favorite doctors, you have made the list."

"Wow, thanks. I'm honored to be chosen. Especially since I'm kind of small potatoes out here. I'm surprised to have made the cut."

"Well, let's just say I have a soft spot for the little guy or gal," she divulged with a wink.

I thanked her again for the information and sample and was walking her out to the optical/ reception area when Dora motioned me over in a panic.

"Good to see you, Ally. Take care," I said as I hurried over to Dora. "What is it?"

"It's the father of Mike Stableson. You know, the high school football player patient who you suggested should take a break from football."

"Oh yes. What's the matter? Does Mike have an eye emergency?"

"I don't think so. But Mr. Stableson is very angry and demands to speak to you about his son."

I took a deep breath and took the receiver. "Hello Mr. Stableson. This is Dr. Trí."

"It's about time, Dr. Trí!" he barked loudly into the phone.

"If you'll just calm down, I could hear you better. How can I help you?"

"You can mind your own damn business for one thing!" he shouted into the phone. "How dare you tell my son playing football is dangerous. Now he's telling me that maybe he doesn't want to play anymore because he doesn't want to bump his head again and get brain damage."

Mr. Stableson was shouting so loudly I had to hold the receiver away from my ears. I hoped Ally hadn't heard him as she was leaving.

"Mr. Stableson please calm down. It is difficult to listen to you when you're shouting," I instructed trying to stay calm.

"Don't tell *me* what to do either!"

"Mr. Stableson, your son did more than just bump his head. He likely sustained a concussion. That is a serious thing."

"What do you know about it? You're not even a real doctor!"

"I am an optometrist. We are primary care eye doctors. We have extensive education on the optics, anatomy and physiology of the eye as well as the diagnosis and treatment of eye diseases," I informed him defensively.

"I could care less. I'm warning you. Stop filling my son's mind with nonsense," he barked before hanging up.

I was stunned. How could any reasonable person behave that way? I don't know how long I stood there holding the receiver trying to process what had happened. The sounds in the office were just murmurs and faded into the background of the drama in my life. I was pulled back to reality by Dora's voice.

"Are you okay Dr. Trí?" she asked again.

"Not really," I gasped trying to hold back tears now that the initial shock had subsided. "People can be so... cruel sometimes Dora."

"Don't let him get to you Dr. Trí. You're a good doctor. You're just trying to help his son. He's a jerk."

"Thanks Dora. Yes, he wasn't very respectful to me. But it begs the question. If he has no problem yelling at me that way, what does he do to his son?"

Chapter 16

I managed to get through the rest of my patient schedule without any additional drama. I smiled weakly when an older gentleman complimented me profusely and said it was the best eye exam he's gotten in years. That wasn't hard to believe since he was wearing a pair of glasses that had photochromic changing lenses, from about two decades ago. The lens company made several upgrades to their product. In the current version, the transition from dark to clear is significantly faster. The downside is that the spectacle lenses do not become as dark, which some may find uncomfortable in a Texas summer. Even good sales in the optical weren't enough to lift my spirits from the awful experience of Mr. Stableson. And then there was John being stolen away from the office and the rent increase. For me, it didn't really feel like a good day.

I said good night to the staff and went next door to the Chinese restaurant to pick up something for dinner. They weren't packed but there were a decent number of folks dining there for a Monday night. I went to the checkout counter to put in my 'to go' order and got a "hello" from

Mr. Tsao, the elderly proprietor. He recognized me and smiled. After ordering my usual, pork and bean curd for me and General Tso's chicken for Fred, I took out the rent increase notice and showed it to Mr. Tsao to see if he had gotten one too. He looked at it and looked at me, but he didn't seem to really understand what I was asking so he called his daughter over to translate.

"Hello Dr. Trí. What can I help you with?" she asked politely.

"Yes, hello Jing. Sorry to trouble you. We got this notice from the landlord of the center about raising our rent and I was just wondering if you got one too?"

She looked the notice over and then turned to her father and spoke to him in Chinese. They went back and forth for a few minutes before she turned back to speak to me.

"My father says he did get a notice like this but didn't really understand it. He says he's been here for many years and has always paid his rent on time so he thought there must have been a calculation error on the rent increase. He put it away somewhere and doesn't remember where. We will probably talk to the landlord later to make sure there wasn't a mistake. It's too much of an increase."

"I agree. Thank you for asking him."

"You're welcome. Enjoy your dinner," she said as she handed me my order that a staff member brought to her.

I bid them goodnight and drove home. It seems the landlord was either trying to make money by overcharging us or else he wanted to get rid of us. Either way, it didn't seem legal to me, or it shouldn't be. I decided not to burden Fred with it. It may open old wounds.

In the beginning, it had been many long workdays between Adriana and me. I paid her and the staff first and didn't pay myself for the first two years. I was lucky Fred was gainfully employed, but those were rough times. The financial uncertainty weighed heavily on my spirit when I was waiting for patients to walk in the door. As more patients came, we were able to shorten our hours by delegating some of the work to staff, but the financial uncertainty was still always hanging in the air. Competition of every kind made a small independent practice a very small fish in a gigantic ocean. Not to mention on-line options were popping up more frequently too. It was a huge strain on our marriage, but Fred realized it would have been worse for me not to try it than to have me always wondering if I could have done it. I generally handled it all and as long as I wasn't in the hole, we didn't discuss it.

When I got home, I called out to Fred that I had brought dinner and I would leave it in the kitchen for him. He was working on another upgrade project for work, so his stress level was high as well. I decided to call my brother for his advice on my lease situation.

His cell phone rang, and he picked up on the third ring.

"Hello," he answered.

"Hey Vu, how's it going? It's Thi."

"Hey sis, what's going on? Not needing Brianna for another sting operation, I hope. Although she really seemed to enjoy the last one. A free manicure, pedicure, hair color and styling, *and* she got to be the hero. I haven't stopped hearing about it for days."

"Sorry about that."

"No, it's a good thing. I like to hear her happy. I buy her what she wants most of the time, but I guess sometimes what someone really wants is to be useful."

"This is true," I agreed. I guess Brianna wasn't so shallow after all. "She was really helpful to us, but this time I wanted to ask for your help with something."

"Woohoo! I was hoping to get to participate too. What do I get to be? A pretend drug dealer? An FBI agent?" he asked excitedly.

"Um, a lawyer," I said slowly.

"But I'm already a lawyer. That's okay, at least I can play one convincingly then."

"Actually Vu, this is not for any kind of undercover work. I need your help as a real lawyer. It's about my office lease. I got a notice from the landlord that he wants to raise my rent to twice as much. Is that legal? I mean isn't there an incremental cap or something?"

"Oh, you have a legal question," he understood at last with disappointment. "You know I do Worker's Compensation law don't you?"

"Yes, but I'm sure you had to have covered something like this in law school. Maybe in contracts or corporate law or something?"

He sighed. "Well go ahead and send it to me along with your lease and I'll have a look at it. But on feeling, I think he could do it if he wanted to."

"The thing is, I know that the powers that be have been trying to acquire property in the area to expand I-45. They have gotten a lot of push back and protests for trying to do it with eminent domain. I feel like this might be a different way for them to do it. Convince landlords to force tenants out by raising their rent and then buy out the landlords."

"Are you talking about a conspiracy?"

"Maybe. Honestly, I'm just trying to stay in business."

"I have to tell you though, even if that is the case, you may not be able to do much about it. It's the landlord's property. He can run it the way he wants."

"Maybe. But if there's a chance to help myself and the other folks in the center, I've got to try."

"Give me the phone," Brianna ordered in the background. "Hello Thi?"

"Yes, hi Brianna. How are you?"

"I'm great. You know why?"

"Why?"

"Because I'm not stuck in a dead-end business scraping by month to month to make rent. Maybe you should just take this as an opportunity to call it quits. I hear you could make lots more money working at the chain store in the mall."

She had obviously been listening to our conversation.

"Yes, I probably could make more money working at that location, but I would have to work their hours 6-7 days a week. Not to mention constantly be harassed to sell whatever products they want to promote, and therefore be way more miserable than I am now. Thank you for your opinion, but I'll handle my own career," I spouted with annoyance.

"Suit yourself," she replied. "I just know that I give Vu advice all the time and he's super successful."

"Okay, I think it might be time for us to go," added Vu regaining control of his phone.

"Thanks bro," I replied gratefully. "Let me know when you know something. Bye."

I hung up the phone and went to eat my dinner. The misery of dealing with business did little for my appetite. When I went into optometry, I naively thought all I had to do was set up an office with the best equipment, give the best care and all the rest of it would take care of itself. Sadly, there was clearly more to it than that. My phone rang and it jolted me from my wallowing. I looked at the caller ID. It was my mom.

"Hi mom," I answered the phone trying to sound cheery.

"Hi Thi. Are you well?" she asked with concern.

"Yes, I'm fine. Why do you ask?"

"Since I live with your brother now, it's hard not to hear things. I heard Brianna and Vu talking about you. It seems that you are having trouble with your business."

"Nothing to worry about mom. It's just a small issue with the rent. I asked Vu to investigate a legal thing with my lease is all. It will be all right."

"You know when you graduated optometry school, your father and I were very proud of you. But when you started the practice, it seemed to be so much work and then there was the tension in your marriage. I know you want to work for yourself, but do you think this is the right way for you?"

"I like being my own boss mom. I like being able to practice like I want and spend as much time with patients as I want instead of just ten minutes and hurrying them out the door."

"I can understand that, and you are a good doctor because you care. But how can you continue to help other people when you're not taking care of yourself. Maybe Brianna is right, and you should work for someone else. Let them worry about the business part and you just be the doctor."

"Thank you for your concern mom, but the last thing I want to hear is that Brianna is right. When I can't do it anymore, I'll stop okay?" I snapped. I spoke more angrily than I intended. I guess all the worry and emotional stress that had been simmering in me for a while had come to a boiling point.

"Okay dear," she assented and then was quiet for a while without hanging up.

"Was there something else mom?" I asked to make sure she was still there.

"You know, I don't want you to think if you decided not to run your own practice anymore that it is a failure."

"But. It does feel that way. What will people think of me? My staff, my peers," I replied unprepared for this assessment and discombobulated by her statement. I could feel involuntary tears start to run down my face.

"They will think you were brave enough to go for your dream and it didn't work out. So, you make a change and find new dreams. You wanted to be an optometrist to help people. You can still do that without having to struggle with a business. There are other ways."

"Yes, I guess that's true," I conceded chuckling and wiping the tears from my cheeks.

"You are a special person, Thi. Sure, your brother makes twice as much money as you, but that's part of his profession. His job is to get as much money as he can for his clients. He has a talent for it. You have a different talent. You have special insight into people and situations. That's what helps you figure out how to help people when others can't. This includes them being able to help themselves."

"Well, I did go to school to learn how to diagnose and treat people's eyes."

"Oh, I wasn't referring to that. Of course, you are good at the science and healthcare part, but you also help people other than patients."

"Which people?"

"People like Lan, Jaime and even Adriana."

"I don't know if Adriana would agree with that. It seems like I bring her more grief than anything these days," I confessed with self-reproach.

"When she was going through a hard time in her life. You saw that and you helped her feel appreciated and find her confidence by asking her to start your practice with you."

"No mom. She asked me to start the office together."

"You've been promoting that story for so long; you have forgotten how it really happened. No offense to Adriana. She is a hard worker, but how could a person with just a high school degree and no formal training in optics, healthcare or business suddenly become a manager of a private practice? You taught her everything she needed to know."

"I guess I did," I replied. So much had happened, I had forgotten the details. "But she must have wanted to do it or else why would she have agreed to it?"

"Because she trusted you. She was in a bad marriage, but she had no financial security so she felt she couldn't leave. You helped give her the power to stand on her own. You gave her the opportunity to be strong and independent by making her your manager so she could leave her marriage."

I hadn't thought about it that way. Perhaps that is why she stays with me instead of going to work for more money at Dr. Moore's office. She's practical and hardworking and can surely work wherever she wanted. Money aside, maybe the things I do have made a positive difference in people's lives. Mothers. Just when you think you have it all figured out, they swoop in and bring you to tears.

"Thanks mom. I needed that tonight."

"I had a feeling," she replied in that motherly way. "Whenever you doubt yourself, you should remember that was why we named you the way we did. We liked the name Thi Trí because it sounds like the tea tree which has special healing powers."

"I didn't know that. How ironic since that's what I tell people who have trouble saying my name."

195

"Yes, it was that and you also have a birthmark on your stomach that looks like a tree."

"Oh!" I exclaimed pulling my top up and looking at my abdomen. There was a birthmark which was left of my belly button. It had been there my whole life and I was just now seeing it differently.

"Good night, dear," she said gently.

"Good night mom. Love you."

She hung up the phone. She didn't often reciprocate the "I love you". It was a cultural thing. I asked her about it once, but she just said, "You know I love you, why do I have to say it all the time?" My mom. What a character.

"She's right you know," Fred added. He was standing in the doorway.

"How long have you been there?"

"Long enough to get an idea of what you've been talking about. You know you tend to talk loudly when you talk to your family."

"Yeah, sorry about that. They drive me crazy sometimes, especially Brianna. Hey, did you know that my birthmark looks like a tea tree?" I disclosed looking at it more. "I don't see it."

"Yes, I know. You don't see it because you're looking at it upside down."

"I am?" I said as I squeezed and folded the skin of my abdomen around the birthmark. I tried rotating it as well as my head. "Oh yeah, I think I see it now. Wow, my whole life, and I never realized it. You learn something new every day."

"I also heard about your rent situation," Fred revealed. "I may be a computer guy, but I can still discuss life issues you know. Why didn't you tell me about it?"

"I didn't want to bother you. Besides, what about our non-discussion agreement regarding my office?"

"I know we agreed to not discuss our work, but I'm still your husband. You can come to me when you're feeling down. I want you to know I support whatever decision you make. Even if it keeps us from living comfortable, financially worry-free lives."

"Thank you?" I replied and gave him a big hug. "Now let's eat some ice cream. It's been one of those days."

We spent the rest of the evening talking and laughing about anything else other than business and it cheered me up immensely. If only this lighter feeling could last.

Chapter 17

T

he next morning, I left for work in better spirits. I was determined to shake off all the negative events that had been happening lately. I even re-considered going to Eyesight Expo. I could make it a mini vacation since it was going to be in San Diego, and I'd take Adriana too. Lord knows she could use a vacation. Dora could handle booking patients for when we got back, and John could get a break from our disappointed stares to focus on selling and dispensing glasses until his last two weeks with us were up.

"Good morning, Adriana," I addressed her cheerfully as I walked in and continued to my office. I put my purse away, booted up my computer and put on my clinic jacket.

"You're in a good mood this morning. Did Vu give you some good news about the rent? Or maybe Fred gave you some..." Adriana replied as she followed me.

"I spoke with Vu last night," I interrupted her. "He says he'll investigate it, and we shouldn't be too hopeful. But you know, there's always hope."

"So why the happy look?"

"Because I think we need a little vacation."

"I think I heard you wrong. I thought you said despite our potential business killing rent increase, loss of a productive employee and mediocre last financial quarter, you wanted to go on vacation. Please tell me I heard you wrong," Adriana demanded sternly.

"You did hear me wrong," I replied smiling. "I said *we* need a vacation. Meaning both of us. And if it makes you feel better, we'll be working as well."

"Now you have really lost me."

"We should go to Eyesight Expo. That way I can get some continuing education hours done, we can get some freebies from vendors and see what's new in the 'vision biz'. And we can do this all while taking in the sights and sounds of sunny San Diego. What do you say? I know you could use some time away from the office even if it's only for a few days."

"Well...I'm not saying I agree with taking time off, but maybe it would be good to see what's new. Okay I'll go, but won't it be expensive with the room and airfare?" she asked pragmatically despite the smile creeping across her face. We both were very proud of what we built, but the onslaught of bad news lately had been draining for both of us.

"I'm checking on the rates now," I stated while seated at my computer. Fred might not be too happy since we were planning time for a vacation together, I thought, but I'm sure he would understand. "We can pay for everything on the company card since it's a business expense. Looks like most flights are booked up. There's a late flight, and it looks like it's a few dollars cheaper too. The hotel near the convention center has special rates if you're going to the conference," I informed her and pulled the web page up on the computer. "Yikes, it's still pretty pricey."

"I knew it. It was a good thought, but maybe next time," she uttered sadly.

"Don't give up yet. I'll call Lan and see if she'll want to join us, that way we can share a room."

"Why would she want to go to an optometry convention?" Adriana asked. "It's not like it will be a great opportunity for her to get new clients."

"You never know," I replied. "There are plenty of optometrists from the greater Houston area that attend. She's so good at promoting her place. Besides, she's usually open to spending time with her best friend. Especially in a hotel by the beach, in a sunny place that is also not dripping wet with humidity."

"Yes, I guess there's that," Adriana agreed.

I dialed Lan's phone number, and she picked up after the second ring.

"Hey girl," she answered.

"Hey Lan. How's it shaking lady?"

"Like going commando in a skirt on a hot Houston day and feeling a cool breeze."

"That's a visual."

"Sorry to hear about your rent troubles though."

"How did you know about that?" I asked surprised.

"Your mom called me and told me about it. Asked me to give you some business advice. Don't worry, I know better than to do that."

"Ugh how embarrassing. Anyway, Adriana and I were planning on going to Eyesight Expo this Thursday and we were wondering if you wanted to join us for a few days of fun in San Diego?"

"Need me to share a room huh?" she asked bluntly.

"Now why would you think that?" I replied innocently.

"Because that's what happened the last time you invited me to one of these conventions."

"Oh yeah, I forgot about that. Well, we still enjoy your company. It wouldn't be as fun without my best friend."

"Isn't that the truth," she laughed. "Those meetings of yours can be quite the snooze. Sitting in lecture halls, listening to all that science and medicine talk. How can you stand it?"

"It's part of the job. We need to keep up to date on the latest and greatest."

"I suppose," she replied dryly. "I tell you what. Ru's been doing so well that I feel confident about leaving him in charge of the salon. Also, since our little sting operation, I've started a girl doing manicures in the salon too. We've had a good bump in sales last month. So, if you promise we'll get to stroll on the beach and eat at some nice seaside restaurants, I'll be happy to come."

"Agreed. We'll have some good girl time," I promised. "But wait a minute. You're doing manicures in the salon now? What happened to you've got standards and you want to keep your salon a classy place?"

"I've still got a classy place and we only do high end and custom designed nails. Ru saw the equipment from our sting operation and suggested we try it. We've had a lot of interest from men and women. You've got to give the people what they want. Who am I to stand in the way of good business."

"I've heard that business advice before. Maybe there's something to it. Anyway, I'll text you our flight information if you want to go when we go, otherwise you can just meet us there."

"Okay girl. I've got to go now. Talk to you later."

"Later," I replied and hung up. I looked at Adriana who was waiting for the results of the call. "She's in."

"Okay, I guess we're doing this," Adriana declared with suppressed excitement. "I'll let the staff know."

No sooner did she leave the room then my phone rang. I checked the caller ID. It was an old classmate from optometry school, Ann Peregrine.

"If it isn't the illustrious Dr. Peregrine," I teased. "How are things in academia?"

"About the same," she replied. "Not much really changes, at least very quickly. How are you, Dr. Tri?"

Dr. Peregrine worked at the University of Houston, College of Optometry. We were in the same class in optometry school. She stayed on as a resident and then as an associate clinician in the contact lens clinic right after graduation and she's been there ever since. She worked her way up to be Director of the Cornea and Contact lens clinic in record time, which I thought was admirable. I had stayed an extra year to do a residency in Low Vision, but after five years of their rules and restrictions, I had to try life away from school. It was a daunting feeling to leave the comfort of the University, but I felt I needed to spread my wings a bit and for better or worse try to make it on my own.

"I'm doing all right. To what do I owe the pleasure?"

"I was wondering if you were going to Eyesight Expo this year?"

"As a matter of fact, I am."

"Glad to hear it. I'll be there too. In fact, I'll be speaking at one of the lectures."

"You will? I thought you usually go to the Academy of Optometry meeting. That's more academic and basic science focused. This meeting is more industry based."

"I do, and I will, but I was a consultant in a study by one of the contact lens companies. I had to make sure there were no adverse effects from using their new contact lenses which they will be unveiling at Eyesight Expo, so they invited me to present the results."

"Aw, I wish I had known earlier, we could have shared a room."

"Thanks, but the company is paying my way."

"Lucky you!"

"I know. I get a suite and everything."

"I'm jealous. What company is it and what contact lens?"

"It's Genericeye Corporation. Their new contact lens is called Plaintoful."

"You are kidding me. I just heard about that from our Genericeye Corporation representative. It sounds like the contact lenses are basically a re-packaging of one of their old contact lenses to be worn with their new Plaintoful eyelash growing gel."

"I wasn't privy to all of that information from the start, I just did the study on the safety and durability of wearing the contact lens. I found out about the marketing scheme after I had signed the contract agreeing to do the study. I guess they needed some legitimacy in their studies for FDA approval. Anyway, it's done. I got a published study out of it and the University gets some good press from doing an industry study instead of just basic science all the time. So, I can't complain about it now."

"Oh, the almighty 'publish or perish' mantra, eh? That's got to be stressful. Having to teach students, work in clinic and do studies too."

"It's part of the job. It beats worrying about paying rent, staff, and the general headaches of keeping the lights on in a business."

"Touché," I replied. Time to steer clear of that unhappy subject. "Can I ask, since you worked with the company, do you know what the active ingredient is in the eyelash growing gel? It seems a bit questionable to me. A miracle concoction of natural vitamins and growth serum that grows dense eyelashes and stimulates gland secretion for more tear production?"

"That does sound too good to be true."

"My gut tells me it is. Do you think you could find a graduate student with a biochemistry background and convince them to figure out what is in the gel? I'd like to know that it is safe before even telling patients about it."

"I don't have a sample."

"Lucky for us I have acquired such a sample."

"How did you get it if it hasn't been officially released yet?"

"Let's just say I have a way with people. In other words, I got lucky," I laughed.

"You are pretty lucky sometimes. However, I don't think I should get anyone at the optometry school involved with it since we have a relationship with the company. Besides, it would be better if a professional looked at it that knows what they're doing."

"That's true, but who?"

"Someone that works in a lab with the proper equipment."

"Like maybe a professor of biochemistry?"

"Yes, for sure. Know anyone like that?

"As a matter of fact, I do. He's a biochemistry professor at the University's main campus as well as one of my patients."

"Really? What's his name?"

"Dr. Kinder."

"Oh yes. Francis Kinder in the biochemistry department. I've met him before at an intra-campus poster presentation session. He has a bit of a chaotic way about him, but he's quite brilliant."

"Sounds like him. A mad scientist no doubt."

"Do you think he'd do it?"

"He just might. I helped him with his contact lenses, and he was so pleased he told me if I ever needed biochemistry advice, I could contact him."

"Was it that great of an exam?" she chuckled.

"I wish I could say that. It's more that he was in such a state of despair having lost his custom-made gas permeable contact lenses. It was easy enough to re-fit him in some new ones, but he was wracking his brain trying to figure out where the old contact lenses went. They weren't in his eyes or anywhere else in his house. Being such a scientist, he couldn't believe that they would just disappear so I helped him find them and he was so grateful he said if I ever needed a favor I could ask."

"Did you go to his house?"

"No."

"Then how did you find them?"

"I asked him to walk me through the last time he knew he had them. He said he was trying to get them out of his eyes and having some trouble. He was getting so agitated that he decided to just go to bed. The next morning, they weren't in his eyes, and he couldn't find them anywhere. I asked him what he was wearing at the time he was trying to take his contact lenses out. He said his favorite wool sweater. I asked him if he wore his sweater to bed. He said no, he took it off and hung it up. I told him to go check his sweater and lo and behold, there were the contacts. They had fallen out of his eyes and got caught in his sweater when he pulled it over his head to take it off."

"That's brilliant. I would have never thought of that. How do you do it?"

"I try to visualize the situation and the possibilities of what could have happened, then I ask questions to either confirm or disprove my hypothesis."

"You're incredible Dr. Trí. If you ever want to work at the University, I'm sure they'd love to have you."

"I appreciate that. For now, I'll slog it out in the trenches. Anyway, I could write Dr. Kinder an email about analyzing the eyelash gel sample. However, since I don't know much about the biochemistry department and you also know Dr. Kinder, do you think if I brought you the eyelash gel sample, you could get it to him?"

"Sure. Just drop it off to me and I'll get it to him."

"Okay I'll drop it off at lunch today. By the way, was this call just to let me know that you'll be at Eyesight Expo?"

"Oh, I forgot since we got sidetracked talking about the eyelash gel. I wanted to know if you were going to Eyesight Expo so I could invite you to dinner on Friday night. You sent me some patients to take part in the study which was very helpful. So, I'd like to show my appreciation. I asked the company representative if I could invite you and they said yes. Besides I hate going to those industry dinners alone. They can be a little..."

"Dry? Boring? Totally commercial?"

"Well, yes."

"I hear you. I would love to come. Could I also bring my office manager and best friend?"

"Uh, sorry I don't think I could sell that."

"No worries. Had to try."

"Same old Thi. In school you always loved the free dinners from industry representatives trying to schmooze with the soon to be new optometrists."

"I was literally a starving student. I think I got down to 98 pounds that last year when all my financial aid money ran out. Now I'm thrifty because I'm trying to grow a business. Maybe someday I'll break the habit, but probably not until I'm retired and then I'll still have to count my pennies. Oh well, such is my life."

"Indeed. I need to go. See you at the Expo."

How nice. I would soon be going to San Diego with Adriana, Lan and now I'll be seeing Dr. Peregrine too. Maybe all I needed was some positive thinking to get things back on track. Even my morning patients turned out to be pleasant and thankful for helping them to better vision. They all came on time, were focused and attentive during their exams, and paid their bill at the end without much fuss. It was days like this that I remember why I went into optometry, to help people see better and make a decent living too. I didn't even mind the midday traffic when I drove to the optometry school, thirty miles from my practice, to drop off the Plaintoful eyelash gel to Dr. Peregrine. Yes, things were turning around. And then I got back to my practice and walked in the door.

"There's a message for you on your desk," Dora informed me. "It's Dr. Moore."

"Thank you," I replied and headed for my office. I sat down at my desk and looked at the message that said simply, 'Dr. Moore called at 12:00p.m. Wants you to call back

ASAP'. Huh. Call him back as soon as possible. We weren't co-managing a patient. My little consulting project with him was long over. Surely this wasn't a reference call about John considering Dr. Moore was the one that had stolen him away from me. No point in trying to figure that man out. Only one way to find out what this was about. I rang the phone number on the message which was his cell phone. He answered on the third ring.

"Dr. Trí, so good of you to call me back. I guess that lovely receptionist of yours gave you my message. She has a pleasant demeanor. Perhaps she would prefer to come work here with us. We are always looking for employees with good people skills," he suggested.

"I think you've stolen enough of my employees Dr. Moore. After all I did for you, how could you steal John away?" I replied angrily.

"Yes, I do appreciate your help in that matter. And I wouldn't say I 'stole' your former employee as much as gave him a promotion of better pay and the experience of working in a larger and more successful office. Wouldn't you want them to advance in their jobs and reach their full potential? Our schedules are packed with lots to do to keep their day interesting."

"You mean schedules overbooked and employees overworked?"

"I haven't heard any complaints," he countered.

That's because they fear reprisals, I thought.

"Have you called just to boast about how your practice is better than mine?" I retorted tersely.

"Not at all. I'm sorry if you feel as if that was what I was doing. In fact, let me compliment you on how well trained your former staff are. They know their technical duties. We just have to re-train them on their independent attitudes.

That kind of thinking has no place in our practice. We want them to do their tasks and only their tasks when we tell them to do it, every day, like clockwork. They have quotas to meet so that they can get their bonuses."

"That's great Dr. Moore, but if you don't mind, I do have patients of my own to attend to, so if you could get to the point of this call."

"Yes, well about those patients of yours. I heard that you have been having a slow time lately and the patients you do see are not particularly happy with you."

"What?!" I cried in disbelief. "Who told you that?"

"A little bird that flies from office to office with all the gossip," he replied smugly.

Ally the Genericeye Corporation representative I thought. I guess she had heard more than she should have after all.

"Your little bird got her tweets crossed. We're doing fine," I fumed.

"Don't get upset Dr. Trí. I'm calling to say that no matter the recent troubles you've been having with patients or lack thereof, we all go through that from time to time. Or so I hear, I haven't personally."

"Get on with it!" I exclaimed.

"I do think that you are a good clinician, so I'd like to formally offer you a job here at our office," he concluded.

"Really?" I replied incredulously. Of all the nerve, after insulting me with his smugness now he wants me to work for him.

"Now you don't have to thank me, just accept and we'll work out the details later."

"What's the matter? One of your doctors finally got fed up and left?"

"Ouch. No, we're so busy that we can always use more help."

"Are you sure you're not just trying to shut down the competition?"

"Ahem, I think we are big enough to not feel too threatened by you."

"Lovely," I replied sarcastically. "I find it hard to believe you are recruiting me just because you think I'm a good doctor."

"Well, it's true. Also, one of our doctors *is* leaving so we have an opening. Besides, didn't you do a residency in low vision?"

"Yes, I did. I just haven't had enough time and resources to build that subspecialty up yet."

"You could do that with us. We already have a pediatric optometrist and sports vision optometrist so it would be a nice addition to our repertoire."

No wonder he was so good at business. He was good at recruiting talent to work for him and no doubt making him tons of money.

"What makes you think I want to work for someone? The point of having your own practice is to be the boss and build a place that offers great products and services and is something to be proud of for yourself, your employees and even your patients."

"And you've done that, bravo. But let's face it, it's a jungle out there. There is safety in numbers. It is far easier and more practical to work as a group to share resources and have more buying power. It's unfortunate that our profession must juggle between being a healthcare service and commodity. Only the strong will survive."

He wasn't wrong there. The idea of sharing expenses and resources was very appealing. Not to mention having other doctors around to share ideas and back each other up when needed. The conversation with my mom last night chiseled away at my confidence that being in business for myself was the right thing and magnified my considerations for calling it quits. Dr. Moore must have sensed I was considering his offer with my prolonged silence.

"All you would have to do is the doctoring and not have to worry about the business side of things. Think of how happy Fred would be when you have more regular hours. You could have dinner together every night and go on vacation together."

Now he was hitting below the belt. Fred would be happier not having to worry about if I was in the red. But what about Adriana? She has been loyal to me all these years. I surely owed it to her to keep going.

"What about Adriana? I can't just close up shop and leave her out in the cold."

"Bring her along. We can find a place for her here."

"Would it be in a managerial position?"

"We have a new manager Bernice, so she couldn't be a manager."

"She has been an outstanding manager for me. She is reliable, hardworking, bilingual, and loyal. Anything less would be a step back for her and I can't do that to her."

"She is definitely loyal since she has spurned my attempts to steal her for years."

"I wouldn't even consider going anywhere without her."

"You drive a hard bargain Dr. Trí," he sighed. "She can be the optical manager. But she would have to report to Bernice."

"No dice. She would only have to report to you. And she'd have to be paid at least the same as she's been making here."

"How much is that?" he asked.

I told him and I think he might have chortled but recovered by feigning to clear his throat.

"No problem," he said smugly. "We'll even give her a raise."

Now I knew he really was doing so much better than me.

"I'll think about it," I said non-committedly.

"That's all I can ask," he ended and hung up. He was pretty sure of himself.

Adriana came into my office after I hung up the phone. I wasn't sure if she had heard any of my conversation, but she kept quiet about it if she had.

"I checked with the taqueria next door. They got the same letter we got about the rent. Looks like we're all in the same boat. Has your brother found out anything more about if we can fight it or not?" she asked.

"I haven't spoken to him since I asked," I replied. "Let me call him now and check."

I dialed his number. He didn't answer. He was probably busy at work, so I texted him that I needed to talk to him. He called a couple of minutes later.

"Hey sis. I'm swamped today, what do you need?" he grumbled.

"Sorry Vu. I was just wondering if you found anything that might help me with the rent increase from my landlord?"

"I did look into it. I'm afraid this is one battle you can't win. Texas law allows a landlord to raise rent as much as they want after the current lease agreement has expired. If you want to stay, you have to pay."

"I was afraid you would say that." I sighed. "Perhaps all the tenants could collectively protest."

"I guess you could try, but you risk him kicking all of you out together and if that is his intention all along, you would be giving him what he wants faster."

"You're right. Thanks for looking into it."

"No problem. Talk to later," he said hurriedly and hung up.

I felt defeated. I shook my head at Adriana. "Nothing we can do."

"Well maybe we can go back to extending our hours or take on more insurance plans," she suggested.

"There is another option," I started hesitantly. "I just spoke with Dr. Moore. He's offered us jobs at his clinic."

"Really?" she demanded angrily. "After all we've been through to build this place, you're ready to throw in the towel?"

"It's not that I want to, but times are changing. Insurance plans decrease our reimbursements constantly. Online retailers are luring our patients away with cheap prices on junk products that people are willing to purchase. Remember the shut down from the COVID pandemic? Remember the time all the staff quit at once? Now we're facing a practice killing rent hike. It seems like the universe is telling us maybe we shouldn't be doing this anymore."

"It's just that I've invested so much time and effort in this place. Years of my life," she uttered close to tears.

"We both have," I replied reaching out to hold her hand. "You've done a phenomenal job. I couldn't have asked for a better employee."

She pulled her hand away. "That's all I am to you, an employee?"

"That's not what I meant," I retracted. "I meant ... associate. You've been my business associate in this from day one."

"Well then as an 'associate' I should have a say in it," she exclaimed.

"You do. That's why I'm discussing it with you. I haven't made any decisions. If you want to keep grinding it out here, we'll do it. However, Dr. Moore says he'll give you a position as the optical manager with more money than what I can pay you."

"He did? I doubt he'd do that out of the kindness of his heart," she said suspiciously.

"I told him it had to be worthwhile for you, and I wouldn't go work at his office without you."

"You did?" she asked sheepishly.

"I did. So, let's sleep on it tonight and we'll reconvene to discuss it tomorrow."

"I guess it wouldn't be the worst thing with all the bad luck we've been having lately. Sounds like a plan boss," she acquiesced after some thought and recovering her composure.

"Dr. Trí," Dora said coming to my office.

"Yes Dora?"

"That patient you saw the other day, the old man."

"The one that said it was the best exam he ever had?" I asked, remembering the compliment.

"Yeah, well now he says he wants to sue you."

"What!" I exclaimed, shocked. "Why?"

"He said the glasses you gave him doesn't turn dark enough in the sunlight and so they gave him skin cancer."

"Are you kidding me?!" I shrieked.

"I wish I was, but I'm not. Sorry doc," she replied and went back to her station.

"What else can go wrong today?" I moaned.

Sadly, I was about to find out.

Chapter 18

I dragged my emotionally beaten mind and body home after closing the office. Not even some new, positive online reviews we had received recently could lift my spirits. I crept in the door quietly. I was hoping to sneak by Fred and languish in a warm bubble bath for a while to wash away the day and heal my bruised soul. He came in while I was mostly immersed in the bath with only the top of my head above water at the level of my nose. It was symbolically fitting as it was how I was feeling about my office right now.

"Bad day?" he surmised.

"You could say that." I replied weakly.

"Do you want to talk about it?"

"Not really," I replied stoically trying not to be needy before breaking down. "Yes, actually I do."

"I'm listening."

"I found out that the taqueria next door to us also got a rent increase notice which eliminates any argument that our rent shouldn't be increased if no one else's is. Vu told me that I have no legal recourse. Then Dr. Moore called to taunt me with gossip from our Genericeye Corporation representative about our office. He informed me that he knows how pitiful our business has been doing before suggesting I should give up the office and go work for him. Then a patient who one day tells me I'm the greatest eye doctor ever, now wants to sue me because his photochromic spectacle lenses don't turn dark enough. Adding insult to injury, he's also claiming that the eyeglasses gave him skin cancer, which of course is a load of horse manure. He walked in with lesions on his forehead before I even said two words to him."

Fred was quiet and taking it all in before speaking. A very wise strategy honed from the many years of being married to me.

"Wow," he said at last. "That's a lot."

"You think?"

"Yeah. You may want to refresh the bubbles every five minutes. I can light some lavender scented candles in here if you like. I hear it helps to relax you."

"Are you being caring or condescending?" I pouted.

"Caring. I don't know what else to say. The last time I tried to suggest something about the office we didn't talk for weeks. Running your own business is hard and it can take a toll on you and your family. I appreciate that you considered my feelings enough to shorten your hours to eight hours a day and take one Saturday off a month so we can have something of a life together."

"Yeah, the hours we have now usually come after being more secure in the business, but I didn't want to strain our marriage to the breaking point. Heck, Dr. Moore got divorced a year after we graduated. I hear he sometimes has his current wife work the phones at his office and I know many optometrists out there with tremendously successful practices but horrific home lives. There needs to be a balance, but perhaps that's where I went wrong for the office," I wondered aloud.

"No, that's where you went right," Fred insisted looking me in the eyes intensely. "I can understand that sacrificing time from the office for your family could lose you some business, but certainly there is nothing you could have done differently that would have prevented your landlord from raising the rent. And this patient of yours with the wacky accusations of his eyeglasses causing skin cancer, on his forehead no less? He's obviously trying to extort you and it's just bad luck that he landed at your door."

"Maybe so," I sighed. "I'm just torn on whether to give up or keep grinding in the hopes that things will turn around."

The landline phone rang just then, and Fred went to answer it. When he came back, his expression did not portend good news.

"What is it?" I asked.

"Your decision may have been made for you."

"What do you mean?"

"That was the fire department. The center where your office is located, is on fire."

"What?!" I cried incredulously.

"I'm sorry Thi, but that's what they said. You'd better get dressed and we'll go down there together."

Now even my relaxing bubble bath was a disaster. This terrible, horrible, day was turning into an even worse night. I got dressed and we drove down to my office. I had called Adriana on the way down and asked her to meet us there. When we arrived in the parking lot there were about three fire trucks with water hoses dousing the flames that were lighting up the night sky.

217

It looked like the fire had started in the back, since the storefront windows and doorway were about the only things left standing. It was harder to figure out if the fire started in the Mexican taqueria or the Chinese restaurant since both were charred much more than my office was, as if the fire started at both ends and moved inward.

Adriana pulled up just as Mr. Tsao from the Chinese restaurant and Mr. Lopez from the Mexican taqueria did as well. Everyone looked stunned. We all greeted each other and congregated together in solemn disbelief as we watched the businesses, we worked so hard for, disintegrate into smoke and blackened rubble.

"Have the firefighters said what caused the fire?" Adriana asked after recovering from her initial shock.

"We just got here ourselves," I replied distractedly as I stared at the flames in disquietude. "We haven't had a chance to talk to anyone."

A tall, sturdily built man with black hair streaked with grey and a weathered face headed towards us. On another occasion, one might have called his tresses a seasoned salt and pepper. But today soot and debris from the fire stuck to it making it more aptly called, ash. He was wearing a firefighter's uniform and carrying his helmet in one hand and a clipboard in the other.

"Can I help you folks?" he asked with authority.

"We are the tenants," I replied. "Adriana and I own the eye clinic, Mr. Tsao owns the Chinese restaurant and Mr. Lopez owns the Mexican taqueria. Or should I say owned."

"Yeah, these situations are always heartbreaking," he replied sympathetically. "I'm chief Burns with the fire department. And before you say it, I'm aware of the irony of my name."

"Any other time, it would be something to bemuse, but not today," I opined despondently.

"Can you tell us what happened?" Adriana asked wiping away an involuntary tear from her cheek.

"Best we can figure is the fire started about an hour ago. By the time it was reported, and we started working on it, it was raging out of control. We couldn't risk sending anyone inside. We just had to make sure it didn't spread further."

"Excuse me sir. Do you know how it started?" Mr. Lopez asked anxiously.

"Well from a preliminary review it looks like an electrical defect. It started in the walls, but once it got close to the cooking areas some grease on the walls and pots of cooking oil on the stovetops gave it fuel to burn out of control."

"Which business did it start in?" I asked curiously, snapping back into reality.

"That's the weirdest thing, it seems like it started in both ends of the structure at approximately the same time. Adds to the idea that it was faulty wiring throughout the building. The odd thing is that the eye clinic had no trouble other than it got caught in the middle of the two fires. Maybe your contractor insulated the wires better since you use more computers and such. We'll have a more definitive report in a few days."

"So does that mean that responsibility falls on the landlord?" Mr. Lopez queried.

"I'm not an expert in those matters, but I would think so since he's in charge of building maintenance. That's not our area, more of a question for the lawyers and insurance people. Sorry folks. I hope you all had fire insurance because there's basically nothing left."

His final words were devastating. Nothing left of the office that was my home away from home these past few years. All the memories of the struggles and triumphs in my practice flashed before my eyes. I was sure Adriana was feeling the same. I turned to look at her and, in that moment, I could have sworn that I caught a knowing glance between Mr. Lopez and Mr. Tsao. It was but a second. A silent exchange but encoded with a familiar and mutual understanding. Could they have been involved? We thanked Chief Burns for speaking to us and for his crew's hard work.

I had mixed feelings looking at the charred remains of my practice. It was a place where I went to work for six days a week, sometimes seven, for years. Adriana, myself, and my staff toiled away endless hours to build it into a quality clinic for the community. We helped many patients there. We had many laughs and occasionally tears, but it was our business. A source of pride and income. And now it was gone. The thought of that made me sad, but admittedly with all the recent problems of the rent increase and unruly patients, it had become less welcoming. I admit there were days I even dreaded coming to the office, afraid of what fresh heartbreak the day would bring. And now, it was as if the problems had also burned up in the fire. Perhaps Mr. Lopez and Mr. Tsao were also feeling the same way given our mutual rent problems. But would they have gone so far as to destroy the source of their livelihoods?

"Did you notice any problems with your electrical wiring lately Mr. Tsao?" I asked, trying not to sound accusatory but needing to know the truth.

"No understand," he said shaking his head. Somehow, I think he did.

"How about you Mr. Lopez?"

"Not that I can remember," Mr. Lopez replied defiantly. "Anyway, like the fireman said, the problem started in the walls so how could we have known there was a problem?"

"Yes, of course," I agreed smiling weakly. "I'm glad you weren't in the restaurant when this happened."

"Yes, that was lucky," Mr. Lopez stated avoiding my gaze and shifting from one foot to another.

"Aren't you usually here late, to close up?" I persisted.

"We have shorter hours after summer. When the children go back to school, people don't eat out as much during the week."

"That's true," Adriana affirmed giving me a perplexed look.

"How about you Mr. Tsao? Don't you usually stay open until 9 o'clock for dinner?" I asked. "It's just 9:30 now."

"We close early tonight. Family problems," he muttered in broken English.

"I see. But you must have noticed a buzzing sound in the walls or felt some unusual heat before you left. And what about the grease on the walls? Your restaurant is usually so clean. How is it that there were pots of cooking oil left out?"

"What are you saying Dr. Trí? They just lost their businesses. I don't think this is the time to be asking such questions," Adriana challenged me angrily.

We stared at each other and there was a tense and awkward silence. Mr. Tsao furrowed his brows, seemingly displeased with the questioning. He motioned to his daughter to come over from the car. When she arrived, he said something to her in Chinese. She listened, glancing at me periodically.

"We are usually open until 9 o'clock on the weekdays, but we had a family emergency tonight. My mother was not feeling well, so my father decided to close early," she explained plainly.

"I see. Well, I'm sorry Mrs. Tsao is not feeling well. It seems her condition may have saved your family's lives," I concluded.

"Yes, it was very fortunate that we were not here when the fire happened. Thank you for your concern," she said cordially. Mr. Tsao spoke to his daughter in Chinese. "My father says he is feeling very tired now. He wishes you all good luck. We are going home now."

"Yes, perhaps that would be for the best," I relented. "Have a good night."

Mr. Lopez bid Mr. Tsao good luck before turning to us. "I will go home too. There's nothing more to do here. Goodbye."

"But I have a few more questions," I started before being cut off by Adriana.

"Good night Mr. Lopez," Adriana interrupted and then stared at me intensely.

"That's not a very happy look Adriana," Fred noted once they were all gone. "What's wrong?"

"What's wrong is that Dr. Trí here is questioning those two men like they had something to do with this tragic fire that burned down their businesses," she accused, not mincing her words.

"That doesn't seem fair," Fred defended, then wondered. "Were you doing that Thi?"

"I don't know, it's just that don't you think it's a little suspicious that the wiring would suddenly go bad in both their restaurants in similar places, at about the same time? They've been here for years and never uttered a word about anything wrong. No buzzing in the walls, no lights flickering. Not to mention there being cooking oil left out to provide fuel for the fire. Surely, it's a health violation to leave pots of oil out unattended," I posited.

"Mr. Tsao's daughter said they had to leave unexpectedly so maybe they decided to clean it up tomorrow," Adriana rebutted.

"And what about Mr. Lopez? Did he have an emergency too?" I countered. "And it would work out well for them with the insurance if the fire department determines it was faulty wiring as opposed to maybe, sabotage?"

"Wouldn't the fire department see if it was sabotage?" asked Adriana. "And how would they have gotten into the walls to get at the wires anyway?"

"I'm not an electrician, but looking at how badly burned their places are, they could have cut a hole in the drywall stripped a few wires, maybe thrown some water on them and no one would know the difference. The evidence would have burned in the fire. You heard the chief. The cooking oil left out or splashed on the walls would have provided an accelerant for the fire to burn fast and hot. And who would question them having cooking oil in their establishments? Had the fire started in just one business, it might not have been able to burn fast enough to take the whole center down. If I were going to burn the place down for insurance money, that's how I would do it. It's just our poor luck that we were caught in the middle."

"Then I guess it's a good thing they were here, so we didn't have to do it," Adriana muttered, her face sorrowful but stoic.

"Adriana!" I exclaimed in surprise.

"Well, she's right Thi. It does rather work out for you too, doesn't it?" Fred added.

"Fred!" I exclaimed again. "What are you two saying? Are you happy this happened?"

"Of course not. But you can't not see how fortuitous this is. You'll get money from your insurance to cover your losses and the others will too on theirs. Even if Mr. Tsao and Mr. Lopez had something to do with this, at least the insurance money will help them to rebuild somewhere else. Seems like they couldn't afford the rent increase either."

"Yes, but they'll only get the insurance money if it's determined to be an accident and not arson," I pointed out.

"Then don't give them reason to believe that it was anything other than an accident Dr. Trí," Adriana asserted looking me straight in the eyes.

"What are you saying Adriana?" I replied uncomfortably. "Are you saying I shouldn't try to find out the truth? Are you saying I should just keep quiet and that maybe it's time to close our doors for good?"

"I'm saying if I wasn't sure what to do before, this is a sign showing me the way. You said yourself earlier today, we did our best and we built something great, but sometimes it's just time to move on. Don't question anymore. Please for once, just let this one go," she implored.

I usually felt that persisting until the truth was uncovered was necessary, the right thing to do, an obligation even. I would question and search until the answers were revealed. As I looked at the smoking, charred remains of my practice, I felt some of that obligation evaporating as well. No one was asking me or even expecting me to give them an answer so maybe I didn't need to this time. I didn't need anyone's permission. *I* could decide to stop asking and to decide what was right to do. What they said made sense. The fire department seemed satisfied with the explanation. No one got hurt. All the tenants would be able to walk away and start again somewhere else. Heck, even the landlord would be rid of us, which was clearly what he wanted by doubling our rent. Perhaps this time the best thing to do, was to do nothing.

"Okay," I sighed. "You win. I'll call Dr. Moore tomorrow and let him know we're joining his team in a couple of weeks. I'm going to hate that smug look on his face."

"A couple of weeks?" Fred asked, perplexed. "Why the delay? You don't have to give anyone notice of your departure."

"We have to let all the patients know what happened and that we won't be rebuilding but closing our doors for good. Not to mention we need to get their outstanding orders of contact lenses and glasses to them. Oh, how much money are we going to lose on the jobs that haven't gotten picked up?" I moaned.

"Don't worry Dr. Trí. The only things that were in the office have been there for months. I was planning on sending them back to the manufacturers. I don't know why people never bother to pick up their stuff. The recently purchased jobs are still at the labs. Finally, a good thing that they take so long to get done!" Adriana exclaimed laughing.

"Yes," I chuckled as well.

"But that should just take you a few days, not a couple of weeks," Fred persisted.

"We're going to Eyesight Expo," Adriana and I said in unison.

Chapter 19

T

he adage of "everything happens for a reason" never gets old for me. The shock and sadness of my practice burning to the ground was a traumatic event for me. But the stresses of business were also affecting me. Looking in the mirror the last few weeks at my pre-maturely aging face and non-dyed, graying hair, was disconcerting. Today, as I woke up in my hotel room in beautiful San Diego, I felt different. When I looked in the mirror to get ready for the day, I saw a face that looked a little more vibrant, fresher, and even happier. When you are in a heavy situation day in and day out, you become numb or unaware of the toll it takes on you no matter how well you try to eat, sleep or exercise. It's no wonder so many Americans are ladened with health problems. We literally work ourselves to death.

After taking care of the last vestiges of my practice and signing on as an associate optometrist with Dr. Moore, I felt a weight lifted from my shoulders. Although I still felt great sadness about burying the literal ashes of the business I had built from the ground up, it also felt like there were possibilities again. What exactly those possibilities were, I wasn't sure of, but just the feeling of a new beginning was uplifting. I think Adriana felt it too. When we were at the airport last night waiting to board our flight to Eyesight Expo, Lan asked us what we were drinking because we were both so giddy. I guess we just felt unburdened. Adriana said it best when she lifted her coffee cup up and toasted, "to new beginnings".

The pounding on the bathroom door broke my reverie.

"Are you almost done in there, Dr. Tri? We don't want to be late for breakfast," Adriana hollered through the door.

"Yes. Sorry, almost done," I replied. I finished putting on my lipstick, grabbed my suit jacket and exited the bathroom. "We can't miss the complimentary company sponsored breakfast."

"It beats the hotel's complimentary room coffee," Adriana replied flatly.

"Coming Lan?" I asked knowing she wasn't since she was still in bed.

"No, it's way too early for me. You guys enjoy. We can meet up for lunch," she moaned and turned over in bed to go back to sleep.

"Okay, we'll text you. Bye," I told her as we headed out the door.

Adriana and I walked happily to breakfast. We were hungry and knew it should be a good meal since it was sponsored by several of the big optical and pharmaceutical companies. When we got to the hotel conference room, it was mostly full. We grabbed the last two seats at a table and got what felt like a visual inspection from the occupants already seated there. They seemed less than impressed.

"Is it all right if we sit here?" I asked politely.

"Is Roger coming?" a dour faced woman asked an older man sitting next to her. Her conference nametag read "Karen Paine, Office Manager".

"Not sure, but he's late if he is. You might as well take the seats," the man told us bluntly with barely an acknowledgement. He was dressed in a nice suit. His tie was pinned neatly into place with a bespoke tie pin. It was round like a circle most of the way but had an extra small bulge coming out of the side like an eye cut in half longitudinally and viewed from the side. It also looked to be 14k gold. No doubt he was successful.

"Thanks," I replied smiling despite the frostiness.

Ms. Paine seemed annoyed with our presence and returned to eating her breakfast. There were water glasses, plates, utensils, and place settings at each seat. It was a buffet style set up, so I told Adriana to get her food first. I didn't want to risk losing our place in case "Roger" decided to show up.

"Anyone know what the talk will be about this morning?" I asked no one in particular but was just trying to break the ice.

I didn't like awkward silence, but I could deal with it if I had to. There was a lot of throat clearing and clanking of forks and spoons against plates and cups. Finally, a middle-aged Indian woman with an "optometrist" title written on her name tag spoke. Dr. Patel was her name.

"I believe it is about the new eyelash gel from Genericeye Corporation," she offered.

"Yes, it says it on the papers that were put on the chairs," Ms. Paine added patronizingly.

She sat stiffly with her hair arranged in a tight bun. She wore a small, gold-plated brooch pinned to her blazer that indicated 25 years of service at her place of work. The numbers were recessed and affixed on a horizontal line behind a large, open arc like a laser light entering an eye. The initials STLC were also recessed and attached to the horizontal line. It was a lovely piece. No doubt she was proud of the acknowledgement.

"Oh right. I guess it would be good to look at the material first," I chuckled nervously.

She replied with an icy glare and condescending nod. My eyes kept returning to the initial on her pin. Finally, I had to ask her about them.

"Excuse me, but what do the letters on your beautiful brooch stand for?" I asked.

"Southeast Texas Lasik Center," she replied tersely.

"Ah yes, of course. It's one of the largest Lasik centers in the greater Houston area," I stated.

"You mean *the* biggest," the gruff man sitting next to Ms. Paine retorted.

I was a little startled at his brashness. The name tag on the man revealed him to be Dr. Lassiere, O.D.

"Pardon me. The biggest," I agreed smiling politely towards Dr. Lassiere. "According to you," I muttered quietly under my breath.

I picked up the papers that had been left on our chairs and looked them over. I realized it was the same product information that Ally Gallagher had given to me in my office. Looks like the company *was* making a big launch of the product during the convention just as Ally had reported. Good opportunity for a large, captive audience.

"Oh yes, my sales representative told me about it. I even got a sample, although I haven't tried it yet myself," I directed at Dr. Patel since she seemed the most collegial.

"You got a sample?" asked Dr. Patel looking shocked. "You must have a big practice. I was told it wasn't available yet until after the conference."

"Umm, well not so big. In fact, I recently closed my office to join a group practice," I confessed for whatever reason I didn't know why. These people already didn't seem to think much of me.

"That's odd," Dr. Patel said. "I'll have to talk to my sales representative again."

"Did you hear that Dr. Lassiere? That Gallagher woman had samples and she didn't give our office any," Ms. Paine uttered bitterly.

"That scheming witch!" Dr. Lassiere spat angrily. "Always trying to find ways to screw me over. I'll have to make sure to let her know that we don't appreciate her behavior. We may even have to get rid of her for services incompetently rendered."

"Whoa doctor! I'm sure she just didn't have enough. No need to be so angry," I exclaimed. I was astounded by the venom he was spewing. That must have been some incident Ally and Dr. Lassiere had to incite such hatred from the man. Still, I'd hate to be one of his patients.

"I can say what I like, and I'll thank you to keep your opinions to yourself Miss," Dr. Lassiere barked through clenched teeth.

"That's doctor," I countered. "And your language is unbecoming of a professional among other professionals."

He glared at me but remained silent. Thankfully, Adriana came back to our table at that moment with her plate full of food, blissfully unaware of the recent unpleasant events. I rose from the table with my plate and went to the food area. I was so upset that I loaded my plate up with blintzes, bacon, and pastries in every flavor, which I probably would not have chosen normally. I needed to calm down, so I checked my watch for the time. It was probably time to check in with Professor Kinder at the University. He had agreed to analyze the Genericeye Corporation eyelash gel sample I had given Dr. Peregrine to give to him. But first I had to get through breakfast. A speaker had come to the microphone indicating that we should all take our seats. I hurried back to my chair and sat down to eat my breakfast. The sound of my knife scraping across my plate brought disapproving stares from my table mates.

"Sorry," I whispered and started to eat more slowly and quietly.

"Good morning doctors and staff," the well-groomed man in an expensive suit bellowed into the microphone. "We hope you have been enjoying the nice breakfast this morning, courtesy of Genericeye Corporation. Let's show them our appreciation for being one of your sponsors and your one stop for all things contact lens and dry eye related."

The room erupted into a round of applause. I wasn't sure if "enjoying" included the company at my table, but the food was good.

"We are proud and happy to announce that soon we will be launching to the public, Plaintoful eyelash gel and contact lenses. The newest and most revolutionary eye products yet. We are confident that you, our eyecare partners, will support our products, and recommend it to all your patients," he announced in typical salesman hype. "Today we are honored to have one of your esteemed colleagues, Dr. Crookes, present you with a talk about the wonders of our product. Take it away, Dr. Crookes."

"Thank you, Jeff," said Dr. Crookes, speaking in a more subdued manner than the salesman. "Good morning colleagues. It is my pleasure to tell you today about this wonderful new product that is going to revolutionize our industry."

Dr. Crookes was well known in the optometric community. Indeed, he was a ubiquitous name on the lecture circuit. He seemed to give industry talks about everything from eyedrops to eye testing equipment. I personally didn't give him much credence since he saturated the market with his presence. I had to give it to him though, he was a great public speaker. Part doctor, part salesman and large part politician, he could probably sell anything remotely connected to the eye. He was in good form today presenting graphs and charts that really didn't say much beyond what was already known about the structures of the eye and the mechanism of hair growth and tear production. Just as with the product literature, there wasn't much substance to the "studies" that were presented in the talk. The end of the lecture always emphasized the billing aspect to the product and how we could increase our bottom line with some ridiculously unrealistic number. I looked around the room at the attendees. Some were looking on their phones and others were listening as though they were back in optometry school. When the talk ended and Dr. Crookes asked for questions, hands shot up. Some of the queries came from friends of Dr. Crookes. They were not real questions but were more compliments to him. I have no doubt their intention was more to brag about an association with the speaker. Most of the other questions were about how to charge for the product or the cost to us. I raised my hand up and after some time, was called on by Dr. Crookes.

"Yes, I was wondering about the side effects? Will we be able to get some information on the chemical make-up of the ingredients ahead of time?" I asked a little embarrassed by the echoing sound of my voice in the room.

"A great question doctor," Dr. Crookes replied. "Genericeye Corporation is still finishing the write up on the latest clinical trials which will be made available in a few months. But I can assure you it is very safe and effective. As for a list of ingredients, it will be listed as a package insert in the box when the products are ready to ship. Next question."

That was a very savvy way of deferring the answer, although it was somewhat brave of him to give his assurance on the products safety and efficacy before it was even out. Then again, he didn't work for Genericeye Corporation. So, what did it matter to him if there was a problem? It would be the responsibility of the company.

After the speakers were done, Adriana and I got up to leave. There was no point in talking further to our tablemates as they all left quickly in silence and without a glance back at us. I was so glad that Adriana was with me. Although I always enjoyed learning at these conventions, it can be so lonely on your own. Unless I happened upon an old classmate, people usually kept to themselves or their groups.

As Adriana and I walked out of the room and towards the main hall where all the vendors had set up booths, I really wanted to know about the results of the chemical analysis.

"Adriana, I really need to make a phone call and possibly check my emails. Do you mind if we go to the business center before we go to the Vendors' Hall?"

"Sure, no problem. I could check my email too."

We headed to the area set up with computers for attendees to check emails. It was nice that the convention hosts set these areas up. Even though most people have smart phones these days, it is a good place to print out things like schedules of presentations or whatever. I'm grateful for computers, but my eyes still appreciate reading paper too. I dialed Professor Kinder's phone number at the University. The phone rang several times before he picked up.

"Hello, Kinder lab," the voice on the other line answered.

"Hello is Professor Kinder available?" I inquired.

"Hold on, I'll check," he replied and set the phone handle down.

After several minutes, a voice came on the line.

"Hello this is Professor Kinder. Who is this?" he asked.

"Hi professor. It's Dr. Trí, your optometrist. You were helping me out by analyzing the sample of an eye gel. Dr. Peregrine from the optometry school gave it to you for me."

"Oh yes, hi Dr. Trí."

"I was wondering if you had the chance to look at the sample yet?"

"I did. Interesting stuff. There were some typical carrier components, water, carboxymethylcellulose sodium, etc., but there were also some growth hormones in there."

"That's right. It's supposed to make your eyelashes grow. They say it's all natural ingredients. Is there a cause for concern?"

"Possibly, after all anything that induces growth of a cell should be closely monitored. I'm not entirely sure if all the ingredients are "natural". However, as a biochemist, I can say that the ingredients in and of themselves are not toxic. The best way to know for sure of its safety is to test it on actual cells and tissue to observe its effect, good or bad. It's hard to say definitively since I do not have human hair and skin cells samples. A complete analysis would test the interaction of this gel sample on these cells. I do have a colleague who works with animal skin cells. She owes me a favor, so I sent her some of the sample. She sent me her results this morning, but I haven't had a chance to look at it. Tell you what, I'll email it to you so you can have a look yourself."

"That would be fantastic!" I exclaimed emphatically. "I really appreciate your help."

"You are welcome. Glad I could be useful. The new contact lenses are working out great by the way. I love them."

"Excellent. I'm glad to hear it," I replied. "Have a great day."

I was thrilled to finally be getting some real information on this mysterious, miracle eyelash gel. Based on my experience at breakfast, I found it odd that Ally, our Genericeye Corporation representative, gave me a sample of this elusive concoction and no other doctors. Speaking of doctors, I should text Dr. Peregrine to see if she was here yet. But first, to check my email for the eyelash gel data. I checked my phone, but it hadn't come in yet. Should I wait for it or go to the Vendors' Hall and try again later? Just then, my phone buzzed signaling me of a new email. I opened the attachment, but there were too many numbers, chemical symbols, and text to see well on the small screen. I decided to just print it out. Hopefully I won't get caught with such proprietary information. But I wasn't anybody in this crowd, so who would think I had anything of importance? I could feel my pulse quicken and was sweating in my suit waiting for the pages to finish printing. There were about ten pages of dense data. This was not going to be light bedtime reading.

"Dr. Trí are you ready yet? I checked my email twice and read all the internet gossip I can stand. I'm ready to see the Vendors' Hall," Adriana whined.

"Yes, just finished. Thanks for indulging me. Let's go," I replied cramming the papers into my purse. They probably would have fit better in the reusable convention bags we were given, but I didn't want to risk anyone seeing them.

Chapter 20

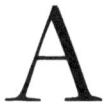driana and I entered the Vendors' Hall and were met with so many sights and sounds. It reminded me of Times Square in New York City. There were hundreds of people talking and milling around. It was a vast space that was simply a single, huge room in the convention center that could be configured to suit whatever group is occupying it at the time. For the Eyesight Expo Convention, every kind of company remotely related to eyecare was there. There were large company signs erected high overhead and hundreds of little booths lined up together along aisles up and down the immense space. The biggest companies had the biggest signs with booths that had multiple, colorful displays and substations for more one-on-one discussions with company representatives. Each company wanted to get your attention and purchase orders, so they had demonstrations of their products, stacks of brochures and, of course, freebies. We usually collected enough free pens to last us all year. Of course, the freebies I really wanted were the sample eyedrops for dry eyes. I liked to have samples for patients to try before they bought the products. These free samples

were not as readily shared by companies. The bigger your office, the more you got. No wonder the folks from the lucrative Lasik Center were annoyed that I had gotten a sample of Plaintoful eyelash gel when they had not. They hadn't even heard of me. I'm sure I did a tenth of the business they did. Oh well, I guess small can also be mighty.

"Where do you want to go first?" Adriana asked.

"That's a good question. Normally I'd want to check out the latest contact lenses or frames that we might want to get for the office, but I guess we don't need to do that now."

"Oh yeah. I almost forgot," she remembered sadly.

"We could find the booths that are having giveaways. Sometimes we can win a smart phone or something."

"That's true. How will we find the ones that are doing that?" she asked.

"It's usually the booth that has the most people around it," I surmised.

"Over there," she directed pointing towards a company that probably made ninety percent of all the eyeglass frames on the U.S. market as well as owning optical chains across the nation and vision insurance plans too. With a finger in so many pies, I couldn't imagine how they could claim to be such a luxe company. Such a monopoly inevitably leads to a decline in quality.

We were making our way over to their booth when a woman who was in a great hurry bumped into me and knocked me to the floor.

"Dr. Trí are you all right?" Adriana exclaimed, reaching down to help me up.

"I think so. Did you get the license plate of that driver?" I joked picking up my bags.

"I'm so sorry Dr. Trí. I didn't see you there."

It was Ally Gallagher, the Genericeye Corporation sales representative. She quickly apologized while picking up some papers she had dropped during our collision.

"Oh, hi Ally. Don't worry, I'm short enough to miss if you're not looking. I'm even more invisible in this crowd."

"Not at all. I'm just in a bit of a hurry," she said nervously looking around.

"Are you hurrying to meet your beau?" I asked.

"My what?" she answered distractedly.

"Tristan Brone, your boyfriend. You mentioned him when we last met in my office that you were meeting him here at Eyesight Expo."

"Oh right," she answered a little flustered. "Well, I, um. We broke up actually."

"Sorry to hear that. I didn't mean to pry into your personal life."

"It's okay. He just wasn't who I thought he was," she opined sadly.

I was about to ask her if she was all right when a company representative for the booth, we were standing in front of, stepped out and corralled us into his area.

"Hello ladies. Might I interest you in a demonstration of our latest slit lamp camera? It can take amazing photos of the anterior of the eye allowing you unparalleled images of ocular structures. You'll be able to capture images of blood vessels, tissue growths, cataracts, lid abnormalities all with amazing clarity and magnification."

"That sounds great. Yes, I would love to try it," I replied excitedly. "But I'll need someone to look at. Would you mind sitting for me Ally? It will just take a minute."

"I don't know," she replied hesitantly.

"I guess I could sit for you Dr. Trí," Adriana offered. "Although I wanted to see the pictures too."

I smiled at Adriana. Out of the corner of my eye, I could see Ally spot someone in the distance and look frightened. She suddenly grasped the seat in front of the slit lamp and sat down.

"On second thought, I'd be happy to sit for you Dr. Trí," she said as she stuck her head in the chin and forehead strap.

"That's the spirit," the salesman encouraged adjusting Ally's head position and fiddling with the camera.

"Uh great," I uttered surprised.

I glanced in the direction Ally had looked and saw Dr. Lassiere. Perhaps wanting to avoid a run in with him could explain her sudden change of heart. Whatever the reason, I was eager to try out the instrument. I sat down on the examiner's side and put my convention bag and purse on the floor next to the machine. I observed Ally's demeanor. She was pale, shaking and taking halting breaths. She looked very frightened, and then she started coughing.

"Do you need a moment to catch your breath, Ally?" I asked concerned.

"Yes," she replied inhaling quick and short bursts of air. "My mouth is so dry. Sometimes it makes me cough. I think I have a peppermint or something in my purse."

She quickly rummaged through her purse, found a piece of hard candy, and popped it in her mouth. It seemed to soothe her for she was able to catch her breath and calm down. After a minute, she stopped shaking.

"Better?" I asked sympathetically.

"Yes, much. Thanks Dr. Trí."

"No problem. Okay, do I have to turn on the camera separate from the slit lamp?"

"Yes, just this on/off switch here. Red light is off, green light is on. Simple," replied the sales representative. "Ms.?"

He asked Adriana trying to read her name tag.

"Adriana," she informed him.

"Adriana, you can look at this computer screen. The slit lamp is sending images to it, and you can see what Dr. Trí is looking at."

I turned on the machine and positioned it so that I had a clear image of her eyelids. The optics on the machine were great. The image was clear and bright, even with the light level on low.

"The image is so bright and clear," I said appreciatively.

"That's because we added extra LED lights on the side bars of the head strap housing to better illuminate whatever you're observing. This gives a better-quality image on the camera since it's not so dark. You can turn them off if you want to just use the central light for posterior viewing," he instructed.

"I see. Yes, that's a good design. Oh, what's this?" I wondered aloud.

I noticed on Ally's lid margins, anterior to the waterline and more on the top lid than the bottom, there appeared to be extracellular growth. It wasn't isolated to a section such as with a pedunculated growth or skin tag, but it went across the whole lid and even started to grow into the tear duct. It was very subtle and a little difficult to see because of the eye make-up. The tear duct is the opening for the drainage system of the eye. The seemingly extracellular growth was most prominent here because instead of growing out, it was growing down into the tear duct. If it continued to grow there, it would block the duct and tears would not be able to drain properly but flow over the lid. No wonder she kept dabbing tears from her eyes in my office.

"Have you noticed any discomfort along your eyelids Ally?" I asked concerned but not wanting to alarm her.

"Not terribly," she answered taking a tissue from the tissue box on the little table next to the unit and dabbing her eyes.

"I don't mean to worry you, but it seems that your eyelid margins have some unusual cell growth. It might be good to have them checked out by a dermatologist."

"Are you referring to the area where my eyeliner is?" she asked.

"Yes. Have you notice it?" I continued.

"Yes, just recently. I had one of the doctors from Genericeye Corporation look at it. He said it was a mild side effect of using the lid gel but that it wasn't anything to worry about because the type of cells growing were typical skin cells that grow there anyway. He said if it bothered me, I could have it removed or cover it up with some make up," she stated trying to sound unconcerned, but the quiver in her voice indicated otherwise. "Anyway, I really must go. I'm supposed to meet with the vice president of Genericeye Corporation at 10:00 o'clock this morning." She looked at her watch. "Goodness, it's almost ten now. It was good bumping into you Dr. Trí."

"Literally," I teased.

"What? Oh yes, right. Sorry again about that. I hope you enjoy the rest of the convention," she said getting up, grabbing her purse, and walking away quickly.

"Was it something I said?" the salesman joked.

"I'm going to say probably not. She said she needed to get to a meeting with her boss. Anyway, I love the unit. I'll take your information and see if my new boss is in the market for a new slit lamp camera."

He happily gave me a stack of information and marketing brochures as well as his card. He thanked us for stopping in and we thanked him for the free pen and yellow contact lens filter.

"So should we try to get to that booth for the smart phone?" Adriana asked.

"It doesn't seem like that crowd has gotten any smaller there. Maybe we should just walk around and then we can think about where to eat for lunch. Lan should be up and about now. Maybe she'll want to join us."

"Agreed."

"I also need to touch base with Dr. Peregrine," I said pulling out my phone.

I texted Lan to tell her where we were and if she wanted to meet us for lunch. She texted back that she would meet us at 11:30 a.m. outside of the Vendors' Hall. Dr. Peregrine said she had to finish up as one of the speakers on a panel and could meet us for lunch if we liked.

"Done and done," I announced.

I attempted to pick up my convention bag. It was heavier than I expected, but probably because of all the paperwork the slit lamp representative gave me. I was about to look into my bag to see what was so heavy when, BAM! I got knocked down again.

"Dr. Trí are you all right?" Adriana asked again.

"Not sure if had fully recovered from the first time," I replied rubbing my shoulder where a tall, slim built, man had pummeled me into the ground. He was neatly dressed in a white button shirt, khaki slacks and a brown tie that was secured with a tie pin. The tie pin was gold colored and featured a round, flat blue stone set in the center with a ring rimmed bezel. Its shape matched the round, gold frames of his eyeglasses.

"I'm terribly sorry. I didn't see you," the tall man apologized offering me his hand to help me up.

The name tag hanging from his neck read Tristan Brone, Ph.D, senior scientist, Genericeye Corporation. I wondered if the tie pin had been a gift from Ally since she was fond of blue.

"It seems Genericeye Corporation employees have it in for me today. I promise I do promote some of your products," I joked as I got to my feet.

"What do you mean? Did you have a run in with another Genericeye Corporation employee?" he asked anxiously. "Because I am looking for one in particular." He said as he moved his head back and forth scanning the area.

"It wouldn't happen to be Ally Gallagher, would it?" I asked, although I was pretty sure I knew the answer to that question.

"Yes, it is. Do you know her? Better yet, have you seen her?" he asked eagerly.

"Yes, some time ago."

"Do you know where she was going by chance?"

"She said she had to go to a meeting with her boss," I answered reluctantly. My gut told me perhaps Ally would rather not see this man, but my instinct to please and be helpful got the better of me.

"Damn it," he muttered under his breath.

"Excuse me?" I replied.

"Nothing," he said flustered. "I just needed to talk with her before she went to see him. Company business. You know?"

"Not really, but I'll take your word for it. Everyone is excited for the launch of the Plaintoful eyelash gel. You're probably glad to see all your hard work pay off," I commented studying his reaction.

"Yes. It's very fulfilling. I'm sorry, but I've got to run. Enjoy the rest of the meeting," he said as he sped off in the same direction that Ally had gone.

I don't think that is going to end well, I thought to myself.

Chapter 21

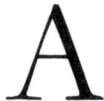driana and I continued to walk around the Vendors'
Hall stopping to watch demonstrations of new products and
picking up samples along the way. Maybe it was my size or
youthful look, but I noticed vendors didn't seem to
approach me as eagerly as my male colleagues. I'll never
forget the time I brought Fred with me to one of these
conventions. He was wearing a name tag that had "guest"
written across it in big bold letters, while mine was labeled
"doctor". Nevertheless, vendors still pushed me out of the
way to get to Fred. The looks on their faces when Fred told
them that I was the doctor, not him, was worth the
disrespect. Especially when I brushed past their apologies
with a look of disdain. Perhaps if I still had my office, I
would be more offended, but today I was happy to just
blend in with the crowd.

At 11:30 we left the Vendors' Hall. It was on the main
floor. I wanted to use the restroom which was on the next
floor up. As we were making our way to the escalator, we
saw Lan at the top of it. We waved at her and motioned for
her to stay there while we came up.

"Hi Lan. Nice to see you up and about," I teased.

"Don't mess with me lady. I barely had any coffee. I don't know who's stocking the hotel room coffee makers, but it's not the best part of waking up."

"The coffee at breakfast wasn't bad. Maybe if you can get yourself up earlier tomorrow you can come with us and get some," Adriana responded sarcastically.

"Umm, no. Still not worth the early wake up. Y'all didn't have to come up. I could have come down, because we'll probably want to get lunch outside of the convention center, right?"

"Sure, but it was no trouble for us to come up. I need to use the toilet and it's on this floor. You want to come with?"

"Sure," they voiced together.

We headed towards the woman's bathroom when we heard a piercing scream, and a petrified woman came bolting out of the lavatory door.

"What's the matter?" I asked stopping her before she slammed into us.

"I think there's a, ... a..." she stammered too afraid the get the words out.

"Spit it out woman. We can't read your mind," Lan said impatiently.

I shot Lan a disapproving look.

"Take a deep breath," I instructed trying to calm her down. She was shaking from fear. "Just tell us what's wrong."

"I think someone's dead in there!" she cried out before fainting to the floor.

"What?!" Adriana and Lan exclaimed in unison.

"You guys are sounding more alike every day," I said. "Take care of her, while I go see if there's something I can do."

A crowd was forming around the woman and people were asking what had happened. Adriana was taking charge and managing the situation like the great manager she was. She was asking people to call hotel management and to help her put the woman in a chair. I was speed walking towards the bathroom with Lan hot on my heels.

"Wait Thi!" she called after me. "You shouldn't go in there. What if there's poisonous gas or something."

"Good point," I agreed and pulled out an N95 mask from my purse and gave her one too.

I continued to keep masks with me wherever I went. Residual habit from the COVID 19 pandemic. You never know what biological contagion was looming around the corner. The mask might not protect me from poisonous gas, but possibly from biological hazards. I figured the lady that ran out would have dropped dead if there was really any poisonous gas.

"Don't you think we should just wait for the police to get here and let them handle it?" Lan asked nervously.

"If the woman is still alive and needs help, waiting could be too late. We must try and help if we can," I insisted. "You don't have to come if you're afraid."

"Who's afraid? I'm not afraid," Lan retorted.

We entered the woman's restroom cautiously. It seemed to be empty.

"Hello." I called out. "Is anyone in here?"

There was no answer except for the echoes of my voice bouncing off the tiles. The doors of the stalls were all half open except for the one at the end of the row that was designated for handicapped. Lan and I looked at each other.

Lan motioned that we should leave, but I shook my head and pointed at the closed stall. I don't know why we weren't speaking. Perhaps the echoing of our voices creeped us out. We moved towards the handicapped stall, and I looked under the door to find a pair of feet on the floor. Someone was definitely in there. I pushed on the door to see if it was locked, but it slowly opened. The squeaking of the stall door as it opened made the hair on my neck stand on end. It was reminiscent of nails scratching on a chalkboard. We craned our necks and peeked into the stall.

"Oh, sweet Jesus!" Lan cried and made a sign of the cross with her fingers.

Sitting on the toilet, fully clothed, and slumped back against the toilet tank with eyes closed and head leaning back as if in a state of eternal slumber was, Ally Gallagher.

"I think I'm going to be sick," Lan announced.

"You and me both," I replied. "Good thing we're in a bathroom. You can vomit in the next stall if needed. I'm going to have a closer look."

"It doesn't look like there's anything you can do for her. Let's get out of here and let the police handle it."

"It's going to be awhile before they get here. We can help them by looking for clues and taking notes of the scene, particularly with the body. Let's see if she's warm or cold, it will give us an idea of how long she's been dead if she *is* dead," I said pulling out my phone and taking pictures of the body and inside the stall before I went into it.

"You're going to touch her?!" Lan asked mortified. "I can't believe you."

"You don't seem bothered when I tell you about all the gross eye stuff I see."

"Yeah, but those people are alive."

I handed Lan my phone and pulled out some disposable gloves to put on. I didn't want to contaminate the crime scene with my fingerprints or catch anything in case she was poisoned.

"Why do you have disposable gloves in your purse? Are you still carrying those from COVID too?" Lan asked.

"No, I got some samples from the vendors downstairs. They're latex free and supposedly softer on the hands. Ooh, they do feel nice," I admired as I flexed my fingers.

"Get on with it!" Lan cried eager to leave.

"Ally. Ally, can you hear me?" I called out to her in case she *was* just sleeping.

My voice reverberated off the tiles. It sounded loud enough to wake the dead. Sadly, there was no response from Ally. The floor in the stall looked clean and dry. Not wanting to contaminate the scene with my shoe prints, I took off my shoes and crept carefully into the stall. The floor was cold, so I was glad I was wearing pantyhose. I admit I probably wore them more for the slimming compression of my abdomen than as a thin sock. I wanted to look professional at the convention.

There weren't any signs of blood or stains on the floor around Ally's body. The walls were clean too. No doubt this was why the non-handicapped, terrified woman, who discovered the body, wanted to use this stall when the others were empty. It's usually cleaner and more spacious than the others.

I observed the position of the body. It wasn't slumped forward or to the side, leaning into the wall. Instead, the body was leaning back with arms pulled together and held there by her clasped hands instead of hanging down on either side. This seemed to indicate that she likely didn't die of a heart attack or stroke. Those deaths would have been more stressful to the person, and I imagine would have been reflected in the final positioning of the body. The current position seemed as if she were simply in sweet repose.

Her blue leather and suede high heeled shoes had scuff marks on the tips and sides. Poor Ally, she loved those shoes. Her clothes weren't disheveled to indicate that she might have been violated, although the top button on her blouse was undone and revealed an oddly shaped bruise on the center of her upper chest below her collar bones. It looked like the partial imprint of a circle. She wasn't wearing a necklace so there wasn't a pendant that could match that shape. Perhaps it might have been from a button, I thought. The ones on her blouse were spherical and made of a pearlescent plastic to mimic pearls so it was unlikely that they were the source. I reached out and felt the side of her neck looking for a pulse. There was no pulse and no breathing. She was still relatively warm and no rigor mortis, so she must have died within an hour or two. Her manicured fingernails were still tidy and there didn't appear to be any blood, skin, or debris under them. There was some faint coloration on her wrists, but the lights might have been playing tricks on my eyes. It's possible she had been wearing bracelets, but there weren't any there now. I opened her eyelids and observed the whites of her eyes had multiple petechia, small broken blood vessels, on them. I took out a penlight and looked at her pupils. They were dilated. A quick look into her mouth and nose revealed them to be clean with no apparent fibers such as if someone had tried to stuff something into her mouth or over her nose to suffocate her. I took my phone back from Lan and took pictures of her head, eyes, the circular bruise imprint on her chest and the scuff marks on her shoes. Finally, I took my gloves off, balled them up and threw them in the trash.

As I put the phone back into my purse and was washing my hands, the door swung open, and a couple of paramedics came in. Lan and I looked up at them in surprise.

"What are you two doing in here?" they asked.

"We came in to see if we could help, but she was already dead," I replied.

"Did you touch the body?" they asked.

"Yes, her neck to check for a pulse. I opened her mouth and looked in her nostrils to see if there were any obstructions and opened her eyelids because they were closed. I wore gloves," I stated. "Are the police with you?"

"No. Why?" they asked.

"Because I don't think she died of natural causes. There are signs that she likely died of asphyxiation although there aren't any marks on her neck. It's possible she was pinned against something that kept her from being able to breathe since there is a mark on her chest. What I am sure of is that she died somewhere else within the last 1-2 hours and moved here. This would imply possible foul play. So, you should have a forensics team in before you contaminate the area."

"Are you some kind of detective?" they asked.

"No. She's married to a policeman," I said pointing to Lan who waved at them weakly. "My name is Dr. Thi Trí, O.D. I'm an optometrist." I stated straightening my name tag.

The paramedics looked at each other perplexed by the situation. Finally, one of them pulled out their phone and called for a homicide detective to come while the other put on shoe covers and went into the bathroom to check on the body. Lan and I motioned that we would wait outside.

Outside the bathroom we both let out a huge sigh.

"What was that?" Lan asked.

"What do you mean?" I replied.

"That Sherlock stuff with figuring out that she died 1-2 hours ago of asphic.., asphiz,.." she stammered.

"Asphyxiation."

"Yeah, that."

"I'm no Sherlock Holmes, just good at looking for clues and imagining a likely conclusion."

"Uh, isn't that what he did?"

"Maybe so, but it seems like all he needed was a few small details and his encyclopedic mind immediately comes to a singular conclusion with no doubt. I look at clues presented, imagine a few possible scenarios, search for lots more information, then present my best conclusion. I guess the key is knowing what additional information to look for. Sherlock was well trained at deductions, I'm good with search engines."

"Call it what you will, it's still something special. And how about the way you talked to those paramedics with confidence and authority. You're not the same unassured Thi I knew back in Houston that would freak out if you had to tell a patient their eyeglasses were delayed."

"I guess I buried that old Thi with the ashes of my practice. I still don't want to deal with irate patients, but I don't fear standing up to them as much. Poop happens, so people need to deal with disappointment. At any rate, I find searching for clues on a dead body is not as stressful as trying to collect service fees from the public. And for the record, that was my first dead body and I hope it will be my last."

"Me too. I'm liking this new confident woman. But tell me, how did you know she was dead for only an hour or two? Or that she didn't just have a heart attack and died?"

"I based the time of death on the fact that the body was not cold yet and no rigor mortis. Besides, I just saw her about an hour or so ago. The asphyxiation was based on the little broken blood vessels on the whites of her eyes. She was likely pinned down because she didn't have any defensive wounds on her hands and arms and no skin under her well-manicured nails. And there was that strange circular bruise on her chest. But it looked like she might have struggled to get out from somewhere because her immaculate shoes, that she was so proud of, were all scuffed up. And her pupils were dilated as if she were terrified. How she was sitting on the toilet made it obvious that she was placed there because her skirt was not pulled up as if she were using the facilities. If she had died of a heart attack, she probably would have been leaning forward or to the side like when you grab your chest in pain. Also, where is her purse?"

"Oh. Well, when you put it like that, it does seem reasonable that she was probably killed somewhere and moved there. Now I see why Jaime likes to pick your brain on his cases."

"Speaking of Jaime, I think you should call him. He can speak to the police when they get here and give us some credibility."

Lan called her husband Jaime on her phone. After a few moments of explanation on her part, complete with raised voices and hand waving, she brought the phone over to me.

"He wants to talk to you," she announced and handed me the phone.

"Hey Jaime, how's the police biz going? Hehe." I laughed weakly.

"You tell me, since you're clearly fond of playing detective," he replied seriously.

"Now I didn't go looking for trouble. It ran into me, in the form of a woman screaming hysterically for help. So, we tried to help, just as you would have."

"I am a trained professional in this type of scenario. From what I hear, you could have just let the paramedics, or the hotel handle it."

"They would have just marched into the area and trampled any evidence, packed up the body and carted it away without a proper investigation."

"Yes, but that's their job. You were supposed to be relaxing at a convention, or at least Lan was. Now you dragged her into a murder scene?"

"That's not fair. She followed me in."

"Don't be cute. I understand going in to try and help if the person was still alive, but once you determined they're dead, couldn't you have just left it alone?"

"First of all, you forget who you're talking to. If I can help, I can't leave it alone. Second, this is personal. I knew this victim. She was my Genericeye Corporation representative. I owe it to her to find out what happened to her if I can."

Jaime was quiet and thoughtful. He let out a sigh of resignation before speaking.

"I know you're right. I blame myself for getting you involved with my cases."

"Exactly," I agreed emboldened. "You let me think I was good at sleuthing. You can't take it back now."

"You do know there's a difference between burglary and murder, don't you? This could get dangerous. I don't want you or Lan to get in over your heads."

"We'll be careful. How much trouble can a couple of little Asian American women get into?"

"Call me when the police get there," he replied with raised eyebrow before signing off.

Chapter 22

L

an looked nervous. She didn't like it when Jaime was upset.

"Was he angry?" she asked.

"Nah. Mostly concerned that we're in over our heads, but I think he wishes he were here helping us."

"That makes two of us."

A crowd continued to linger in our area. I could feel a pair of eyes staring at me. I looked around and spotted Ms. Paine, the office manager at my table during the breakfast meeting looking at me from a few feet away.

"I'll be right back," I told the others and went over to talk to her.

"Hello Ms. Paine," I said cordially.

"Hello Dr. Trí," she replied in kind. "I should have suspected you would be at the center of a commotion. What have you done now?"

"As a matter of fact, I just discovered a deceased body in the restroom. A woman we both know."

"Oh? Who would that be?"

"It is Ms. Ally Gallagher, our sales representative with Genericeye Corporation," I informed her while observing her expression closely.

"Really? So, she's dead then?" she inquired coolly.

"Yes. You don't seem very surprised," I replied astonished at her dispassion with the situation.

"Well, I saw her earlier today near that restroom as a matter of fact. She was standing outside of it coughing and wiping her eyes profusely. I approached her and asked if she was all right. She replied that she just needed to catch her breath. I noticed that her eyes were watery and red so I thought she might be having problems with allergies. As I also suffer from allergies, I had some medication in my purse. I offered her a tablet. I see now that the problem was something else."

"How long ago was that?" I probed.

"Maybe about an hour ago."

"Karen!" a thundering voice called.

We turned to see Dr. Lassiere coming up the escalator.

"Where have you been? I thought you were just going to go to the restroom."

"I was, but it's been closed off. I guess I'll have to find a different one."

"Did you take care of things?" He lowered his voice and glanced at me.

"Yes. It's all done."

"Great, then let's go."

They walked off without another word to me. They were an interesting pair. He seemed easily provoked and she was ever so discreet and steady.

"Coming through!" A voice commanded as a couple of uniformed policemen arrived along with a man dressed in a plain suit. I surmised him to be homicide detective based on his authority.

The paramedics had come out of the bathroom and were detailing the situation to the detective as one of the officers was putting up yellow caution tape and the other was dispersing the crowd.

Adriana and the woman who found the body made their way over to us just as the paramedics were pointing in our direction.

"What's happened?" Adriana asked.

"It's Ally, our Genericeye Corporation representative. She's dead," I informed her sadly.

"Oh my god!" Adriana exclaimed.

"Excuse me. I'm Detective Henderson. Are you the optometrist?" Henderson asked me as he approached us.

"Yes sir. That's me, Dr. Thi Trí, O.D. at your service. I suppose you want to know some information about the patient, I mean victim," I corrected. "Sorry, force of habit."

"Actually, I want to know why you two were in the bathroom alone with the victim when the paramedics arrived," he questioned combatively.

"Well detective, after this woman ran out of the bathroom in a panic and yelling that someone in the bathroom needed help. We, as good Samaritans, went in there to see if we could be of assistance. Are you implying we had something to do with her death?" I rebutted firmly.

"I'm just trying to understand why two random people would willingly go into a place where a deceased person would be if they did not have anything to do with that deceased person to begin with."

"First of all, we didn't know for sure that she was dead. So once again, we went in to see if we could help," I stated bluntly. I could feel my blood pressure rising.

"That's right. That's what happened," the woman with Adriana said.

"And who are you?" he asked curtly, turning to the woman.

"I'm Fiona Oglesby. I'm an optometrist attending this conference and I was the one who first found the body when I went into the restroom to use the toilet."

"You're an O.D. too? Nice to meet you Dr. Oglesby, I'm Dr. Trí. Do you practice in the area?" I asked collegially putting out my hand.

"Yes, my practice is in San Diego," she replied shaking my hand.

"Now stop that!" the detective snapped. "Okay so you weren't in there initially, but after you determined Ms. Gallagher was dead, why did you stay take it upon yourself to touch the body and make observations such as, 'deceased likely not dead from natural causes, but asphyxiation. Possibly by foul play'?" he asked, reading from his notes. "Fancy yourself a detective, do you?"

"I fancy myself a concerned citizen with an earnest desire to help someone I knew," I countered. "We stayed to make observations and gather clues from the scene before it became compromised. We knew the deceased because she was our Genericeye Corporation representative. We wanted to help her in any way we could. I took pictures of the stall before I entered, and of the body which I will gladly share with you. There are signs of foul play judging from the broken blood vessels in the whites of her eyes, dilated pupil, and an unusual bruise on her chest. It's circular as if it might have been made by a pendant or a button, or a…"

"A what?" he asked impatiently. "What are you looking at?"

"A tie pin," I gulped. "That's a nice tie pin you have on detective."

"Thanks, it was a gift. Is that all?"

"Um, no. We saw the victim over an hour ago, alive and without a mark on her. Additionally, her shoes have scuff marks on them which were also not that way earlier."

"Here you are Officer Henderson," Lan said handing him her phone. She had quickly called Jaime again. "My husband is with the Houston police department. He can explain to you."

"That's Detective Henderson," he corrected as he took the phone from Lan and walked away to speak with Jaime in private.

"Thank goodness we called Jaime ahead of time," I whispered to her.

"And thank goodness he picked up," Lan added.

"Okay so your story checks out. You are who you say you are," Detective Henderson said more calmly as he returned to us.

"Good. I can send you, my pictures. Would you like us to help you compile a list of suspects, because there are a few I can think of," I offered.

"No. You've done your civic duty and now it's time to leave it to the professionals."

"But we can help. You'll want to know who had a motive to hurt her. She had an ex-boyfriend who works at the same company. He bumped into us earlier today. He was chasing after her and seemed upset about something. Maybe a lover's tiff, or maybe something about work since she was headed to see their boss. And then there was one of her clients from the Southeast Texas Lasik Center. He is a very unpleasant man. He was steamed that she didn't give

261

them samples of the new eyelash gel ahead of time. Even threatened to get rid of her," I rattled off.

"I don't think anyone would kill for a sample of eyelash gel."

"It's a hot ticket item. They're unveiling it tomorrow and seems like no one has gotten a sample."

"Except you," Adriana added.

"Yes, well except me," I said quietly aware that it was proving to be more of a suspicious gesture than I initially thought.

"And so how did you acquire this exclusive item?" Detective Henderson asked, perking up at this tidbit of information.

"Ally, the sales representative and deceased victim, gave it to me. She said she thought I was a good doctor and wanted me to evaluate it. I guess she valued my opinion," I proclaimed defiantly, but now wondering myself.

"Very well," he acquiesced. "Here's a card with my contact information. Give me all the information you have, particularly for this ex-boyfriend. He seems like a more likely suspect. We'll have to wait for the medical examiner's report to make sure there was even foul play. You'll excuse me if I don't take your word on cause of death."

"Absolutely. I specialize in eyes, not dead bodies. Perhaps you could let us know the results of the M.E. report? Please," I requested in the most charming voice I could muster short of batting my eyelashes, which I might have done unconsciously.

"You really are nosy, aren't you? We'll see. Officer Jaime said you might have insight into the case. Since I don't know you, you'll forgive me if I'm more skeptical," he stated less contentiously.

He thanked us for the help and told us to stay away from further police business as he left.

"Well ladies, thank you for helping me out earlier but I think I'll be going now," Dr. Oglesby said.

"Yes, not your standard introduction. It was nice meeting you. I hope finding a dead body didn't spoil the convention for you," I replied.

She half smiled and walked away.

"I hope finding a dead body didn't spoil the convention for you?" Lan asked sarcastically.

"I didn't know what else to say," I replied. "I felt like it needed to be acknowledged."

"Optometrists are weird," she said shaking her head.

"Just this one," Adriana chimed in.

"Okay, no more pile on. I liked it better when you two were making fun of each other instead of me," I complained.

My phone buzzed and I looked at the caller ID. It was Dr. Peregrine, so I answered it.

"Hi Dr. Peregrine."

"Hi Dr. Trí. I'm done with my lecture panel. Are we still on for lunch?"

"Lunch, uh sure. We're finishing up with a situation here. Would you mind meeting us at our hotel room? It's next to the Convention Center. Room 2022."

"Sure, I'm staying at that hotel too. Should I go there now?"

"Yes. We'll see you soon. Bye."

"Bye."

"What do you mean meet us at our hotel room? I just came from there. Aren't we getting lunch?" Lan asked.

"I just want to put my convention bag away, it's really heavy. Also, Dr. Peregrine did some consulting work for

Genericeye Corporation. We should tell her about Ally's death. And maybe she can tell us more about the ex-boyfriend to see if he's capable of murder," I mused as we walked to our hotel room.

"Oh no. I know that look. You're not going to let this go, are you Dr. Trí? Didn't you hear what Detective Henderson said. He told you to leave the rest to the police," Adriana ordered.

"He said to stay away from police business. That means paperwork and telling people what to do. We're going to try and find out who did this, how and why. For Ally. She deserves to have the truth revealed," I proclaimed.

"Lord help us when she gets like this," Lan bemoaned.

"No kidding. Especially since she doesn't have a practice to keep her preoccupied," Adriana added.

We hurried back to our hotel room. When we got there, Adriana headed to the bathroom.

"I'm glad we came back to our room. I've been needing to pee for hours," she said.

"Why didn't you go when we were standing right next to a restroom?" Lan asked her outside the bathroom door.

"Because I had to take care of that lady who fainted, and I didn't want to pee near a dead body."

"Makes sense," I replied. "Gosh what is so heavy in my convention bag?"

I emptied the contents of my convention bag onto my bed.

"How many pens did you get?" Lan asked laughing at my collection.

"Listen, I just lost my business not too long ago. Don't judge me," I said as I sifted through the items. "Pens and eyedrop samples don't weigh much. It must be all this paper. I don't remember getting all this material."

I picked up some paperwork and looked through it. It was not brochures and advertisements for companies but instead looked like proprietary company reports. There were pages of data and analytics. After a few moments of sifting through the pages trying to figure out why and how these papers got into my convention bag, I finally found a page that had highlighted areas and notes written in red pen ink that said, "proof that gel causes cancer!". Another page was a copy of a memo from the vice president of Genericeye Corporation to the company's lead scientist. It read, "Don't release this data publicly. Results are not definitive. Keep it under wraps until more testing is done. We will go ahead with public unveiling and get the product out now. We need to start recouping money for all the research and development of the new eye gel.".

"Holy crap!" I cried.

"What is it?" Lan asked.

"This is proprietary company information about Genericeye Corporation's new eyelash gel product and it's not good. According to this data, not only do the growth hormones in the gel cause growth of eyelashes, but it also causes excessive growth of skin cells."

"Is that bad?"

"If it was just a few normal cells maybe not because we're constantly shedding some when we wash or rub our skin, but this shows that the growth is abnormally disproportionate to that and can possibly lead to those cells turning malignant. Meaning cancer."

"Are you serious?"

"And the worst of it is that the company's head scientist and vice president know this but are keeping quiet about it and releasing the product anyway."

"How did you get this information?" Adriana asked, coming out of the restroom.

"It must have been Ally. When she bumped into us at the Vendors' Hall. She was carrying a bunch of papers. She must have put them in my bag in case something happened to her."

"And something sure did," Lan said shaking her head from the memory of discovering the body.

There was a knock on our hotel room door that made us all scream with surprise.

"Who is it?" I asked tentatively.

"It's Dr. Peregrine. Are you ready for lunch?" Dr. Peregrine asked through the door.

"What should we do?" Adriana asked anxiously. "I'm sure you are not supposed to have these papers and if Dr. Peregrine worked for Genericeye Corporation, wouldn't she have some loyalty to them? She could confiscate the papers and they would get away with everything. Even murder."

"True. She's more of a 'toe the line' type of person and defers to her superiors, but she has a strong moral compass. I trust her." I decided after some thought. "We'll let her in and tell her what's happened. She can help us. We'll figure it out together."

I opened the door for Dr. Peregrine and motioned her inside. She looked confused by our secretive and somber faces.

"What's going on? Did something happen?" she asked carefully.

"Yes, looks like my hopes for lunch in a nice restaurant by the beach is not happening," Lan moaned.

I threw a pillow at Lan, and it hit her in the face.

"Ow. What was that for?" she grumbled rubbing her forehead.

"This is serious Lan," I admonished. "We'll order room service, okay?"

"That works I guess," she sighed.

She went over and sat down at the desk in the room. She started looking at the hotel's restaurant menu. Even though she didn't want to show it, I could tell she was anxious because eating soothed her.

"Why are we not going out to lunch?" asked Dr. Peregrine.

"You'd better sit down," I said solemnly and pulled a chair over for her. "By the way, this is Adriana, my office manager and Lan my best friend."

"Hello," they said in unison.

She sat down and we told her about the company papers and finding Ally's body and our theories for a murder and cover up. She listened quietly. The shock of the events left her speechless. When we were done, she stayed silent for a long time.

"So, you think, this Genericeye Corporation representative was killed because she threatened to expose the company's research on the Plaintoful eyelash gel?" she asked at last.

"We don't know for sure," I answered. "She never told us anything about it, only why else would she put these papers in my bag? The problem is, we don't even know if she made it to see the vice president. Her ex-boyfriend was hot on her heels in the Vendors' Hall. It's possible he found her first and silenced her. We were wondering if you could tell us more about him. What kind of person he was. If he would be capable of murder."

"Wow, that's a big leap to make," she contended. "But how can you be sure this data is even legitimate. Maybe they're doctored or misinterpreted. No offense to your friend, but she was just a salesperson. Did she really know how to read scientific data?"

"That's a good point," I concurred. "I have something that might tell us."

I pulled out Professor Kinder's colleague's data sheets from my purse.

"Do you remember the Plaintoful eyelash gel sample I had you give to Dr. Kinder at the University to analyze for me?"

"Yes," she replied.

"I have the results. Dr. Kinder emailed it to me this morning. I haven't had time to look at it, but it is an independently tested, unbiased analysis. Let's see what it says."

I looked through the papers. Most of the information were lists of sample size, analysis times, chemical components, and descriptions of cell samples. I flipped through the pages until I came to one that stated, "Conclusion: More long-term testing needed, but preliminary results indicate gel sample uses artificially synthesized hormone components to activate and extend growth cycle of hair and skin cells indefinitely while simultaneously inhibiting normal factors that would stop the cycle. Continued growth of the cells would promote mutation and possibly lead to malignancy".

"This is it!" I exclaimed. "Read this."

I handed the papers to Dr. Peregrine. She looked over the report.

"So that's what you were printing out this morning," Adriana concluded. "No wonder it took so long."

"Why did you have the gel analyzed yourself?" Lan asked.

"I figured with all the miraculous claims it was making, it had to be too good to be true. I wanted to make sure it was legitimate before I recommended it to patients."

"That's why she's my eye doctor," Adriana stated proudly.

"But how can you know for sure that the papers are hers and that she knew what was happening at the company?" Dr. Peregrine questioned again.

"I recognize the writing of the notes on the papers. It looks like her writing. I think she also thought something was off so she purposefully gave me the sample knowing I would probably test it. She wasn't giving the samples out to every office and was a little secretive with it when I think about it. The last thing she said when she gave the gel to me was, 'use it wisely'. What else could she have meant by that? I sat at a table of very angry optometric people at breakfast that didn't get anything for their much more successful offices."

"As long as we're throwing around theories, do you think one of those people from breakfast could have killed Ally?" Adriana asked.

"They did seem pretty put off by the perceived snub, but I agree with Detective Henderson, I can't see not getting a sample as enough motivation for murder," I replied.

"What about if an affair with one of those people, caused them to have a very nasty divorce?" Adriana speculated. "That might be a motivation for murder."

"Who did that? And how do you know about it?" I asked confounded.

"I hear things," she said smugly. "You doctors think you're the only ones that interact with each other. Staff talk to each other too, especially if there's juicy gossip about the doctors. It was that Dr. Lassiere at the Southeast Texas

Lasik Center. He had to pay out a truck load of money to his ex-wife. And after his divorce, Ally dumped him and went on as if nothing happened. His staff says every time she would come by, he was in a bad mood. Sometimes he would mutter about getting her back."

"Yes, that would be a pretty good motive. He even threatened to 'get rid of her' at breakfast this morning, in addition to some other words I will not repeat. He certainly seems to have enough of a temper to do it. How long ago was this?"

"Probably about a year ago."

"Something to consider."

"This all seems so unbelievable," Dr. Peregrine declared. "I worked with this company for months. They all seemed so professional and positive. I can't believe I didn't see any of this."

"Well, you saw what they wanted you to see. Besides you only worked with the contact lenses. You had limited exposure to the eyelash gel, which is what they wanted I'm sure," I figured.

"But medical malfeasance, cover ups, murder? You must admit, it's too much to believe!" Dr. Peregrine exclaimed. "Before we jump to conclusions, how do you know she intentionally put the papers in your bag. Maybe it was an accident."

"Does it really matter if it was. That doesn't change the data, or the company's intent to deceive the public for money," I countered. "Greed and corruption are real and dangerous things. I'm sure Genericeye Corporation has invested millions of dollars in research and development for this product. They are not going to let anyone get in the way of their bottom line. No offense, but you've been living in the sheltered world of academia. It's a jungle out here in the world of free enterprise. Where the competition is always a few paces behind you and profits and losses are the only things that matter for your survival."

Dr. Peregrine's face dropped in a pained expression. Perhaps I went a little too far, so I dialed it back.

"Besides, she was very nervous when we bumped into her. Due to the importance of these papers, I highly doubt she would have let them out of her sight. In fact, she said she was on her way to talk to the vice president. Perhaps they were going to talk about the clinical results, or else she might have been planning on confronting him," I hypothesized.

"Oh damn, he was the one that killed her!" Lan shouted.

"Shhh!" Adriana, Dr. Peregrine, and I shushed Lan together.

"Sorry, I mean he has to be the one that killed her if he was the last one to see her alive," Lan whispered.

"But we still don't know if he was the last one to see her alive," I asserted. "Besides there is something else to consider. Ally had a circular bruise in the middle of her upper chest. There aren't many things that can make a mark like that. I think it might have been from a specially shaped button or tie pin since they would be about the right size and position depending on the person's height. Remember how her ex was trying to track her down. He was very emotional, and he had a tie pin on. It's possible he got to her before she even met with the VP."

"That's right!" cried Lan. "He did it. He's got to be the one. He hunted her down and hugged her to death. It was a crime of passion."

"That's one serious bear hug," Adriana interjected.

"But we can't be sure of that either," I considered. "Did you see how scrawny he was? And if you're looking for a crime of passion, Dr. Lassiere was very passionate in his contempt of Ally. He had a tie pin on too. The circular shape would fit exactly."

"So, he's the killer?" Lan asked impatiently.

"Except that, given his size and temper I imagine there would have been a huge fight. He might well have snapped her neck if given the chance. Considering that she didn't have any bruising anywhere else on her body, or any indication that she fought back. That's confounding," I contemplated aloud.

"Is this how you are when you're trying to figure out what's wrong with your patients?" Lan joked.

"Uh, kinda. You can't just throw a diagnosis down when the signs and symptoms aren't clear cut. You need to look at differentials to eliminate what something couldn't be as well as considering what it could be."

"If you're doing all that, how do you actually finish an exam on time?" Lan teased.

"Sometimes she goes a little long," Adriana chimed in. "Trust me though, it's only because she wants to get it right."

"Aw, thanks for understanding that, Adriana," I said appreciatively. "And here I thought you were always mad at me for going over time on my exams."

"Oh, I don't like it. Especially when I have to hear all the complaints about how long you're taking, but I get it."

"Okay, so you're careful. But in this case, have you had enough time to think about it yet? Who do you think did it?" Lan asked fervently, wanting the answer.

"I don't know yet," I replied. "There are too many suspects and too many possible scenarios. It's all muddled. I know there's an answer, we're just missing something. I need to get into my subconscious."

"You need to do what? How are you going to do that?" Dr. Peregrine asked.

"I don't know. Usually when I'm stuck on something, I do something quietly distracting like crocheting or knitting. It preoccupies my waking mind while my subconscious mind is still working on the problem, and it usually helps me to solve it. Afterwards, in addition to the answer, I'll also have something nice like a scarf or mittens. Sometimes it even comes to me when I'm sleeping in the form of an odd dream or something. I need to quiet my mind and visualize what might have happened. Anybody have that meditation app on their phone?"

"Why don't you just look out the window? Aren't we near an ocean?" Adriana asked.

"Unfortunately, a room with a nice view would have cost more," I replied regretfully.

"How about if we talk about some of the lectures going on at the convention?" Dr. Peregrine asked, always the academic.

"I think that might be a bit too intellectually engaging," I replied to her disappointment.

"What about a game?" Lan asked feeling bored.

"I don't know if I'll be very good at that. I get anxious with timed competitions," Dr. Peregrine replied nervously.

"You do research. Don't you have a timeline on when you need to get data and write papers?" I asked.

"That's different. I'm only competing with myself then. And I usually have months to years to do it."

"Don't worry. It's all for fun. A light-hearted distraction," I reassured her.

"Let's play charades. I'm first!" Lan exclaimed.

She got up and motioned that it was a person. Then started to make stabbing and strangling motions.

"I'm going to guess a murderer," I said dryly.

"You got it," she replied. "Now tell us who it is."

"Very funny," I countered. "You're not helping."

"Sorry Thi, but I'm starving. You promised me that we would have nice meals by the seaside, and I haven't had one yet."

"You're right. Why don't we go ahead and order some room service," I suggested. "Also, I have come to a conclusion."

"What is it?" Lan asked eagerly.

"We need more information. The answer feels very close, but we can't get it without knowing all the facts. Rest assured. We'll get there, ladies."

"What do you mean *we'll* get there?" Dr. Peregrine asked.

"Oh boy, here we go again," Adriana uttered rolling her eyes.

"What is she talking about?"

"What she's talking about is that Thi is too deep into this now. She is going to investigate this thing until she gets an answer or gets herself killed, and probably the rest of us too," Lan wailed.

"I think you're getting 'hangry', Lan. You're clearly overreacting," I declared.

"Is she right Dr. Tri? Are you going to endanger yourself and your friends by pursuing this investigation rather than leaving it to the authorities?" Dr. Peregrine questioned with a reproving look on her face.

"All I'm suggesting is that we help the authorities by gathering up evidence wherever or to whomever it leads so that they can catch the culprit. For Ally's sake, and might I add for our sakes too. Can you really say you feel comfortable being at this convention with a murderer running loose? We know more about this than they do and even if they believe our theories, which at this point they probably don't, it will take them too long to get to the evidence before the convention is over and it's too late. If we can get some hard evidence against the killer, then they can do their job. Without enough probably cause, they can't even get a search warrant. Isn't that right Lan?"

"Hey, I'm not the cop in the family. But based on years of listening to Jaime working, I think she's right," Lan agreed.

"And if in the process of gathering evidence of the murder, word leaks about the dangers of the eyelash gel, well the public has a right to know that as well," I added.

"But that's proprietary information," Dr. Peregrine protested.

"Normally I would agree with you, but in this case it's a public safety issue. It is your responsibility to share what you know about an ocular product if you know it will harmfully affect someone. Remember the oath we took as optometrists, 'I WILL advise my patients fully and honestly of all which may serve to restore, maintain or enhance their vision and general health'. Not to mention, 'I WILL do my utmost to serve my community, my country and humankind as a citizen as well as a doctor of optometry'."

"Is she always this passionate about healthcare?" Dr. Peregrine asked Adriana.

"Why do you think I'm still willing to work with her," she replied.

"Very well," she sighed. "Tell me what I can do to help."

"That's the spirit," I cheered. "We'll have to see if we can question her ex, but first I need you to tell me about who this VP is and then we need to find a way to get into his office alone to snoop around for evidence." The color seemed to drain from her face. "But let's have some lunch first."

Chapter 23

L

unch from the hotel room service wasn't half bad. My chicken salad sandwich had walnut and cranberries in it which perked up my spirits. Sometimes it's the little things in life that help get you through the day. Although we had to eat in our hotel room, the view out of our window showed a blue and clear sky.

"So how much do you know about the Vice President of Genericeye Corporation?" I asked between bites of my chocolate chip cookie.

"You can read his biography on their website for education and work history specifics, but Mr. Colin Cooper is as ivy league as they come. He has a bachelor's degree in Biochemistry from Stanford and an MBA from Harvard. His father started a fortune 500 company and I think his mother comes from money. Genericeye Corporation brought him on a few years ago to help with new product developments. Given his family pedigree, I think he has something to prove. He is cordial but aloof. He keeps his thoughts close to his vest. And they're nice vests too. He's usually always dressed in three-piece tailored suits and polished Italian leather shoes. I've never seen someone dress so fancy every day of their life. He probably doesn't even own a pair of jeans."

"Does he wear tie pins?" I inquired.

"If he's not wearing a vest. Most of the time he will tuck his tie into his vest. My favorite one has round, flat buttons that look like black opals set in a smooth, gold bezel. It's so chic."

"Indeed," I replied picturing the size, shape, and position of where the buttons would be on the vest.

"He also has an impressive collection of cufflinks. Lots of jeweled ones in just about every color to match his mood. We usually knew if he was in a good mood if he wore his green, emerald pair. If he was in a bad mood, he'd wear his black onyx pair."

"Did you meet with him often?"

"I've only met him a couple of times but talking to some of the scientists with the company, everyone is intimidated by him. Can't say he was that impressed by me, but I figured I was too small a player to show up on his radar. He is going to be at the dinner tonight. You can meet him yourself."

"That will be useful, yes, but since his name is on this incriminating memo, I don't think he's going to be forthcoming in our investigation. I think the only way we're going to get any answers is to get into his room to see if there are any signs that Ally made it in there," I hypothesized and tried to imagine what I would even be looking for.

"How are we going to get into his room? I'm sure there will be plenty of security. In fact, the whole floor is probably off limits since they have a block of rooms reserved for all their company employees."

"We'll need a distraction," I said looking at Lan and Adriana.

"Excuse me, why are you looking at us?" Adriana asked in her sassy Latina voice.

"Oh, I thought I heard you volunteer," I replied with a mischievous smile.

"Dr. Trí, you're a great eye doctor, but you need to get your hearing tested."

"Come on girls. This is your chance to showcase your finest acting skills."

"Did I say I wanted to be an actress?" Adriana replied. "This is way above my pay grade."

"First of all, I've seen your acting for the last five years when you pretend that you are so happy to help those patients who want to try on all the frames in the optical and then decide to use their old frames. I mean it is academy award material. Secondly, undercover operations are fun. Tell her Lan. That sting we set up at your salon was so fun I still smile when I think about it."

"Oh yeah," Lan replied sarcastically. "I loved losing a morning of business so I can set up a fake nail salon and be treated like dirt by women with too much money."

My searing gaze sent a chill down her spine. She got the message.

"But really Adriana. It was so fun. You can pretend to be someone completely different. Why don't you pretend to be an overly controlling Latina woman with a big chip on her shoulder and an even bigger mouth," Lan laughed.

"What?" Adriana exclaimed indignantly. "Then why don't you pretend to be a wardrobe challenged, talks-too-much Asian woman with clown colored hair because she's colorblind."

"Oh no you didn't," Lan snapped standing up and coming face to face with Adriana as the two of them lock eyes in the ultimate stare down.

"Ladies, ladies," I interjected separating them. "I think both of you would play those characters wonderfully."

"What!" they cried in unison.

"I mean, they're characters after all. Not who you really are, right?"

"Right," they agreed in unison.

"Okay so hug it out and let's get the plan together."

They approached each other slowly and when they were within arm's length, reached out and patted each other on the shoulder and then went to their separate corners. With goodwill mostly restored, we spent the next hour working on how we would draw any security away and how Dr. Peregrine and I would get into Mr. Cooper's room.

"But how will we be able to open Mr. Cooper's room door once I've identified it?" Dr. Peregrine asked.

"Are you very good at pick pocketing? Perhaps you could get his room key out of his pocket and slip it to me as we're passing each other?" I suggested.

"Pardon me for using such terminology and no disrespect to the mentally ill population but are you insane?" she exclaimed.

"Possibly," Lan said.

"Definitely," Adriana added.

"Maybe just a little," I acknowledged. "I like to think of it more as being imaginative, embracing the possibilities, …"

"Please Dr. Trí come up with something more steeped in reality. There is no way I will be able to get close enough to Mr. Cooper to steal his key, nor would I be able to pull it off. Know your limitations. I know mine," she declared firmly.

"Okay fair enough," I acquiesced. I paced the floor thinking of how we could do it. The minutes ticked by, and we would lose our opportunity if I didn't think of something fast. I was focusing so hard, I found myself staring at the wall without blinking which made my contact lenses dry out. Blinking profusely and hit with inspiration, I suddenly ran over to the door of our room and opened it. Then I examined the door lock, handle, and door frame. The others watched me with a mix of fascination and skepticism.

"I've got it!" I exclaimed.

"Tell us," Lan asked eagerly.

I picked up my purse and rummaged through it until I found what I was looking for.

"When Mr. Cooper opens his hotel room door, you can stick this single, disposable contact lens flat pack into the mortise in the door frame. Bubble side inward of course. That way the door will close but not lock."

"What the heck is a mortise?" Lan asked.

"It's the hole in the doorframe that the lock fits into."

"How in the world do you know that?"

"Because I broke one once moving furniture into my house. It's a long story, trust me on this."

"And how do you propose I get it to stick there?" Dr. Peregrine asked.

"With this!" I showed them excitedly pulling an object out of my purse. It was a small, rectangular strip of double-sided tape.

"What in the world are you doing with double sided tape in your purse?" Adriana asked.

"What *don't* you have in your purse?" Lan joked. "No wonder it's so heavy. Do you have an umbrella that you fly around with in there too?"

"Don't be ridiculous, I would totally use a jet pack. Solar powered of course," I quipped.

"Naturally," Lan replied.

"Ahhh!" Lan and I laughed and bumped fists.

"Can we get back to the issue at hand?" Dr. Peregrine interrupted impatiently.

"Right. Sorry. I usually carry some with me to conferences and conventions to remove lint off my clothes. I may not be much to look at, but I am a professional."

"That makes total sense," Lan concurred.

"Anyway, keep the contact lens flat pack, pre-loaded with tape in your jacket pocket and when you get close enough to the opened door frame, stick it in there. Then while you and the Genericeye Corporation folks are headed down to the distraction that Adriana and Lan will so skillfully provide, text me his room number. I'll do the rest."

"You make it sound so easy," Dr. Peregrine wailed.

"It won't be, but I have confidence that you can do it. Just visualize yourself doing it. Swallow your fears and go for it."

"I'm not as fearless as you are in these situations Dr. Trí," Dr. Peregrine expressed, brows furrowed with worry.

"Oh, I think you're more capable than you think, and you've got better credentials too. You graduated top of our class while also doing additional research projects in clinic and being student representative for our class. You gave a poster presentation at the Optometry Academy meeting while still a third-year student. I couldn't have done that. In fact, I finished somewhere in the middle-ish ranking in our class, and grateful that I got through school. So, you got this Dr. Peregrine."

Dr. Peregrine looked at Lan and Adriana who returned her gaze with smiles and thumbs up gestures. She smiled weakly back at us and then nodded.

With each person's task defined, we synchronized our watches and smartphones, and split up to our respective parties. Dr. Peregrine and I headed to the twelfth floor where Genericeye Corporation's employees' rooms were and where their temporary office quarters were located. She would request a meeting with Mr. Cooper under the guise that she needed to check how the new contact lenses were being presented along with the launch of the Plaintoful eyelash gel. This would justify her presence on the floor allowing her to visually scout out the physical whereabouts of Mr. Cooper and anyone else on the floor, including security.

It was past two o'clock. Luckily, most of the employees would be out setting up the evening's program for the official launch of the Plaintoful eyelash gel. It was go time.

Chapter 24

D

r. Peregrine and I rode the elevator up to the eleventh floor together. I would get out at the eleventh floor and take the stairs up one more flight. Then I would wait for her signal to enter when it was all clear. In the elevator I could sense Dr. Peregrine's uneasiness by her rapid breathing and dilated pupils.

"Are you going to be able to do this?" I asked her.

"Yes. Sure. I'm just having a mild anxiety attack. It will pass I'm sure," she heaved holding her hands on her hips and trying to take deep breaths.

I pushed the stop button to halt the elevator.

"What are you doing?" she asked anxiously.

"I'm pressing pause on this operation until you are calm and collected enough to do it. If they figure out what we're up to, we might end up like Ally."

"Oh god. I don't think that's helping," Dr. Peregrine said hugging herself and pacing around the elevator box.

"I'm sorry. You're right. That was insensitive of me," I apologized rubbing my forehead and feeling my heart rate increase as well. "Okay, what usually calms you down when you're dealing with an unruly patient in clinic?"

"I usually stop what I'm doing, whether it's typing on the computer, at the phoropter, or looking in the slit lamp. I put everything aside and look at the patient quietly."

"What? Do you mean you just give them a hard stare?" I asked, intrigued.

"Yes," she replied confidently. "I sit on my stool quietly and I look at them, not angrily, but calmly until they've stopped ranting, crying or carrying on."

"And that works?"

"Sure does. You can fight with someone who is shouting or fussing at you, but you feel uncomfortable if someone is just quietly staring at you. If you really want to discombobulate them, raise an eyebrow for a disapproving look. The combination unhinges them or at least it makes them nervous enough to stop and ask me what I'm doing."

"And what do you say?"

"I say their behavior is not helpful to me when I'm trying my best to help them with whatever it is they came to see me for."

"And then what happens?"

"If it's a reasonable adult, they apologize. If it's a child, they get intimidated enough and calm down. In either case I carry on."

"How often does that work?" I asked amazed and unsure if I had the inner steel for that.

"Most of the time. The unreasonable adult or medically problemed child are told to reschedule until they can control themselves."

"Wow, maybe working at the optometry school isn't so bad after all. Sounds like patients are beholden to you and not the other way around."

"Don't get me wrong, the College needs patients to train students with as well as their fees, but patients have access to very well-trained doctors and all the latest equipment there. Plus, we have the luxury of not overloading our exam schedules so patients can be sure they will get great care. Therefore, it behooves them to do their part and behave during an exam."

"Amen to that. Okay well doctor, just think of this situation as dealing with an unruly patient. Only the patient is the vice president of a huge corporation, and your goal is to convince him to leave his room for a short period of time. Be dispassionate and firm. Look him in the eye when you are speaking, believe what you are saying, and no one will doubt you."

It took me a long time to learn that this was the way to get most patients to get over my petite size and youthful appearance and see me as a competent healthcare professional.

Dr. Peregrine's breathing relaxed, and her pupils returned to normal, standard illumination, size. She seemed calm and ready to go so I pushed the button on the elevator to resume our upward course. When we got to the eleventh floor, the elevator stopped, and the doors opened. I gave Dr. Peregrine an encouraging nod and wished her good luck as I got off the elevator and headed towards the stairs.

When Dr. Peregrine reached the twelfth floor, she squared her shoulders, lifted her head, and walked out of the elevator doors towards the block of reserved Genericeye Corporation rooms with confidence and a singular purpose.

"Whoa, there Miss," said a large man in a security uniform stopping her abruptly. "This floor is off limits to the public. Only Genericeye Corporation employees are allowed."

"Yes, I know," she assured him. "I work as a consultant for them. Here's my convention badge. If you look me up, you should find me in the company roster as a consultant. I'll wait."

The security guard was so surprised by her confidence, he almost let her through.

"Okay, stay here and I'll check," he said as he pulled out his walkie talkie.

"Hi Dr. Peregrine!" a man in a light colored, summer suit exclaimed waving at her from the hall. His conference tag indicated that his name was Aaron Merica, an employee of Genericeye Corporation. He had just walked out of his room and saw her with the security guard.

"You know this woman?" the guard asked.

"Of course. This is Dr. Peregrine. She's been working with us to get FDA approval for our new contact lenses. What are you doing here?"

"I came to talk to Mr. Cooper about how the new contact lenses were going to be launched with the Plaintoful eyelash gel this evening. Is he available?"

"Uh, I'm not sure. He's very busy. I saw him a few minutes ago. He was taking a phone call in his room."

"Okay, I can go over some details with you if you have a minute."

"Sure, I was about to go down to the Vendors' Hall, but we could talk for a bit."

"Okay ma'am, but just stay with this gentleman and keep clear of Mr. Cooper's office."

"Whatever you say," she smiled. "Wouldn't want to do anything illegal. But which room is Mr. Cooper's. So, I can stay clear of it."

The guard pointed it out to her, and Dr. Peregrine nodded and smiled. She and Aaron walked off together down the hall.

Dr. Peregrine went with Aaron into one of the rooms next to Mr. Cooper's. He swiped the door with a hotel card.

"Is this your room?" Dr. Peregrine asked.

"Oh no, this is a common room for all of us. We have group meetings here."

"That's a good idea. You can have more privacy from the convention attendees to go over company strategies and all. How often do you all use this room? Is Mr. Cooper in his room all the time?"

He looked a little unsure of what to make of her questions.

"I'm just curious. I would imagine he would have to hear all the chatter and it would make it hard to sleep," Dr. Peregrine stated calmly.

"Oh right," Aaron agreed relaxing. "I don't think the noise bothers him. He likes to hear that we're working. Besides I doubt if he even sleeps much. He's really wound up about the Plaintoful launch. Also, he's got a suite which is huge. It doubles as his office here. He'll pull someone in there for a private meeting if he feels like they are underperforming," he whispered the last part.

"I'm sure you haven't been in there," she smiled awkwardly.

Aaron looked at her, unsure if she was flirting or not. Dr. Peregrine looked around the room. There were several cases of Genericeye Corporation's medication samples stacked against the walls.

"Wow. Are these cases all samples the eyelash gel and contact lenses?" Dr. Peregrine asked.

"Most of them. There are a few samples of our other pharmaceutical products too. We don't just do eyes."

"Really? I didn't know that, of course I guess I mostly pay attention to eyes. What are they for and why are they here?"

"They are cough medication and antihistamine tablets. It was cheaper to ship all the sample products here together. The local Genericeye Corporation sales representatives for the non-eye products will swing by and pick them up to take on their routes to doctors' offices in the area. I'm glad I only do the eye products. It's less complicated and lighter to carry than the regular medications. Just between you and me, I think it's pretty genius that the company who makes medications that help dry you out from colds and allergies, also makes eye drops for dry eyes. Getting paid for both sides," he laughed.

"Yes, that is something," Dr. Peregrine laughed in agreement. "It makes sense if you are doing all the research and development into medication to solve several problems at once. More cost effective."

"Exactly. And profitable."

"Yes, of course. Deadlines must be pretty tight sometimes."

"Absolutely. I've seen them filming commercials for products before they even get the final okay on the last clinical trials. Time is money."

"Wow really? I guess I can understand that. I bet they would lose a lot of money if they had a targeted launch date but got held up on a product because the product didn't do everything it said it would or had bad side effects."

"Oh yeah. That happened with our last cold medication. Apparently, it was too powerful and caused significant dehydration in people. It even caused respiratory distress in people with predisposed respiratory illnesses like asthma and such. It cost them several millions of dollars to reformulate. But you didn't hear it from me. Now what did you want to tell me about the contact lenses?"

"Well," Dr. Peregrine started trying to think up a convincing enough reason for being there when suddenly we could hear the guard's walkie talkie outside of the door and the guard responding that he will let Mr. Cooper know.

"I wonder what's going on. We should find out," Dr. Peregrine directed.

"After you," Aaron said motioning to the door. Dr. Peregrine put her left hand in her jacket pocket and held the contact lens pack loosely in her hand while making sure the sticky tape, bubble end was facing away from her palm. They came out into the hallway in time to see the security guard knocking on Mr. Cooper's door.

"Mr. Cooper sir," the guard called through the room door.

The door opened and Mr. Cooper poked his head out.

"Yes. What is it?"

"Sorry to bother you sir, but there seems to be a disturbance at the Genericeye Corporation booth downstairs."

"What kind of disturbance?"

"Two women are complaining loudly that the new eyelash gel is a fraud. They're saying they want to see the company's senior leadership about it."

"Christ that's all we need. Okay I'll come down," he uttered annoyed. He turned and spotted Dr. Peregrine and changed his demeanor. "Oh hello. Dr. Peregrine, is it?"

"Yes, hello Mr. Cooper. Good to see you again," she said positioning herself in the doorway so that her back was against the open doorframe.

This forced Mr. Cooper to take a step back since she was so close to him. Dr. Peregrine stuck her right hand out to shake Mr. Cooper's hand and distract him from noticing her left hand pushing the contact lens flat pack into the mortise of the door frame. Mr. Cooper shook her hand awkwardly.

"Yes, well I would like to chat, but I have a situation happening downstairs, so I have to go down to the Exhibit Hall."

"It sounds dreadful. We'll go with you," Dr. Peregrine offered and motioned for him to go forth.

Confused but in a hurry, Mr. Cooper went first, followed by Aaron. Dr. Peregrine made sure the door to Mr. Cooper's room closed gently so as not to dislodge the contact lens pack. She then started to follow the others when she stopped at where the security guard was standing.

"Shouldn't you be coming too?" Dr. Peregrine instructed the security guard.

"What for?" he asked.

"In case these women start a physical altercation with Mr. Cooper. They could be animal rights fanatics against the animal testing on the products. They can get violent I hear. Besides, no one else will be here and the rooms are all locked."

"I guess you have a point," he agreed and followed them to the elevator.

Dr. Peregrine followed, quickly texting me Mr. Cooper's room number.

As soon as I got Dr. Peregrine's text, I opened the doors of the stairwell and walked into the twelfth-floor hallway. It was quiet and deserted. I hurried to Mr. Cooper's room scanning the hallway with my eyes left and right cautiously. When I came to Mr. Cooper's room, I put on some hand-crafted, knitted gloves I had made and brought from home.

I was sad that I only had one pair of those rubber gloves from the vendor, but happy that my crafting skills came in handy. I didn't want to leave fingerprints. I gently pushed on the door of Mr. Cooper's room. The door didn't budge. Oh no, I thought. Maybe the contact lens didn't stick to the mortise and the door locked. I was frustrated, so I banged on the door, and it jiggled. I pushed the handle down and pushed hard on the door and it opened. Hallelujah! Our plan worked after all. I just needed to push harder. Timidity will get you nowhere apparently.

I opened the door carefully and looked around to make sure there weren't any security cameras around. It looked clear so I walked in, pulled the contact lens pack out of the mortise, and slipped it into my pocket. Once inside, I closed the door. The room was tidy. The bed was made and devoid of clothing, papers, and the like. Everything on the desktop was neatly arranged. Mr. Cooper seemed like a man that liked order. There didn't seem to be any signs of a struggle. I went to the trash can by the desk and saw a discarded tissue that was marked with traces of make-up. There were also a small, torn piece of plastic sealant and a discarded bottle of eye drops. I recognized the bottle as the same one that Ally had pulled out of her purse at our last meeting in my office because it was covered in make-up. I bent down and picked up the bottle and shook it. It still had liquid in it. I opened it and took the cap off. There was mascara around the collar of the tip. It was the same bottle. So, Ally *was* in the room. I pulled a plastic bag from my purse and put the bottle, the plastic sealant, and the tissue in it. The bag didn't have a self-sealing component at the mouth of it, so I tied it shut with an elastic band and stuffed it into my purse. While I was near the ground, I noticed some dark scuff marks on the floor in front of the desk. I pulled my phone out and took pictures of it. Then I enlarged it and noticed that it had some blue coloring to it. It was the same blue coloring as Ally's shoes. I held my breath with excitement. This was an indication of a struggle. In fact, she may have even been killed here, I thought. I jumped with a start when my phone vibrated. It was a text from Dr. Peregrine saying they were on their way up. I rushed to the door and left the room. I moved to the other side of the hallway and started looking at room numbers as the elevator doors opened and Mr. Cooper, the security guard and Dr. Peregrine came hurrying down the hall.

"Who are you and what are you doing here?" Mr. Cooper demanded loudly.

"Who me?" I replied innocently. "I'm Trí. Dr. Thi Trí, O.D. I'm here for the eye conference. Who are you?"

"I'm Mr. Cooper the vice president of Genericeye Corporation and this is a restricted floor."

He really did look every bit the well-groomed power executive that Dr. Peregrine had described. Not a hair was out of place. Dust seemed to float away from his expensive tailored suit and fancy shoes as if not daring to soil his perfect ensemble. His tie was neatly tucked in place. It didn't need to be kept immobile with a tie pin since the bespoke vest with the fancy, round buttons did the job just fine. His cufflinks were shined up and sparkling with the look of success.

"Oh, I'm sorry. I didn't know that. I was just looking for Dr. Peregrine. She told me she was stopping by."

"Yes, this is my old classmate Dr. Trí. We were in optometry school together. She helped to recruit patients from her own practice for us during the Plaintoful contact lens study."

"Hm, did she?" He responded more calmly. His gaze was steadily fixed on my face as if gauging my threat level. "Thank you for your contribution, Dr. Trí, but it would be best if you didn't come up here again. After all, if you found out our company secrets, we'd have to kill you," he said adding a menacing smile to imply he was jesting, but not really. The unblinking severity of his gaze was frightening.

"Hehe. Good one," I replied weakly and swallowed hard. "Well Dr. Peregrine if you're all done here, we should be going."

"Yes, we need to get ready for the Genericeye Corporation Plaintoful eyelash gel and contact lens launch dinner tonight. Dr. Trí will be my guest."

"I'm very excited about the product. Ally Gallagher is my Genericeye Corporation sales representative. She's great. I mean she *was* great since she was found dead today. A very sad thing. Are you familiar with her?" I asked observing his expression carefully.

"Hm, Ms. Gallagher," he replied putting his hand to his chin and ruminating as if trying to recall the name and the person. "Oh yes, I'm familiar with her. I did hear something about her death. Terrible thing her passing so suddenly. She must have had some hidden health problems."

He spoke affectedly as if trying to project compassion. However, when he noticed my scrutinizing stare, his demeanor changed back to simmering annoyance.

"What do you know about her death?" he asked. He was hovering over me, using his size advantage as an intimidation tactic.

Time to be provocative.

"Well, I was passing by this morning when I saw them taking her body out of the restroom where she was found,"

I stated calmly. "I'm curious by nature, so I spoke with the investigating detective. He wasn't sure what she could have died from. The thing is, she seemed perfectly healthy to me when I bumped into her this morning. So, I suggested they pay extra attention to any toxic substance in her blood or stomach that might have killed her. Perhaps she was given something that stopped her breathing. But what do I know? I'm just an optometrist."

I stood my ground in front of him and matched his gaze. He didn't blink or flinch at my words. We stood there staring at each other, locked in silent psychological combat.

"Okay, so we're going to go now. We'll see you at the dinner tonight," Dr. Peregrine said pulling me away.

We walked towards the elevator, and I could hear Mr. Cooper admonishing the security guard for leaving his post. When we got into the elevator and the doors closed, I let out a huge sigh of relief.

"What was that all about?" Dr. Peregrine asked breathing easier as well.

"I just wanted to see what his reaction was when I mentioned that Ally was dead. I'm feeling like he's the murderer," I declared.

"What? He is the Vice President of the company. Why do you think it's him?"

"Because if the eyes are the windows to the soul, I've had a look in and the devil has made himself at home."

"Okay that's dramatic and a little dark. But tell me, why would he risk murdering her and how would he even do it?"

"I think we've established the why, I just need to figure out the how."

"You didn't tell me that you suggested the detective pay attention to any toxic agents in Ms. Gallagher's system?"

"That's because I didn't."

"Then why did you lie about it?"

"I was bluffing hoping to get lucky. I wanted to see if he would react to it. Besides, while I was in his room, I found these," I said pulling the bag that contained the tissue, plastic sealant and eyedrop bottle from my purse and showing them to Dr. Peregrine.

"A used tissue, a shard of plastic and an eyedrop bottle?" she replied unconvinced.

"They belonged to Ally. I bet they will have her fingerprints on them proving she was in the room."

"Okay, but even if they were hers, you can't definitively prove it was her that put them there. Perhaps she gave them to her ex-boyfriend, and he threw them away there."

"I guess that's a possibility. But I also found this!" I declared and showed her the picture of the scuff marks on the floor I had found.

"What is that?"

"They are scuff marks from Ally's shoes. You can see the blue coloring. So not only was she in the room. I believe she was killed there. She struggled against her killer who probably had her tied up or something, so she couldn't get away."

"Well, if they did have a physical struggle, it doesn't seem like it was too difficult for Mr. Cooper. His appearance was as immaculate as ever."

My eyes welled up with tears at the thought that Mr. Cooper's menacing eyes were the last thing Ally saw as her life was taken from her. She needed justice. I needed to give it to her.

We hurried back to our room where we found a voicemail waiting for us on the hotel phone. We played it. It was Detective Henderson saying he had Adriana and Lan with him in the business office of the convention hall and that we should go there to collect them.

"Oops, I forgot to tell you. It slipped my mind since I was distracted by the epic stare down going on between you and Mr. Cooper. Hotel security detained Adriana and Lan for their diversion stunt. They were going to call the police to arrest them for disturbing the peace, but then Lan suggested they call Detective Henderson instead. I had to act surprised about the whole thing, so I left them there and went back up to the twelfth floor with Mr. Cooper. We probably should go to Detective Henderson right away to get them," Dr. Peregrine suggested.

We rushed over to the business center where Adriana and Lan were sitting quietly and a little worse for wear.

"Detective Henderson. Thank you so much for coming to our aid," I cooed as sweetly as I could.

"You women are certainly a handful. What's this all about?" he asked with a bemused expression.

"We discovered some incriminating corporate paperwork that shows Genericeye Corporation's new eyelash gel product could cause abnormal cellular overgrowth of the eyelid," Dr. Peregrine explained.

"And this is bad?" Detective Henderson asked, raising his eyebrow inquisitively.

"Yes, detective. In layman's terms it means that their eyelash gel could create tumor like lesions on the eyelids. But instead of stopping production and investigating this, they are planning on launching the product now anyway and not telling anyone. My Genericeye Corporation sales representative, and recent homicide victim Ally Gallagher, knew this and was trying to confront the vice president about it. That's where she was headed this morning when she bumped into us in the Vendors' Hall. We now know that she *did* see him in his room and that he most likely killed her to cover it up," I revealed passionately.

"Wow, really!" Adriana and Lan exclaimed in unison.

"You girls have really got to stop doing that. It's a little unsettling," I said.

"My sentiments exactly," Detective Henderson agreed. "Not what you said. What they said. How did you get these company papers, how do you know she was in his room and what proof do you have of this '"murder"?'"

"Just before Ally saw Mr. Cooper, she ran into me in the Vendors' Hall. Literally ran into me, knocked me down and everything. It's not unusual given my size, but honestly how hard is it to look down occasionally."

"Get to the point," he interrupted.

"Right, sorry. She told us that she was heading over to speak to Mr. Cooper after we were trying out a new slit lamp camera where I looked at her eyelids and saw this extra cellular growth for myself. In fact, we need to go back to that booth and get a copy of those pictures before they delete them!"

"Later. Continue," Detective Henderson directed sternly.

"Well, she must have figured her meeting would go badly because she put the company papers in my convention bag which we found a few hours ago. Also, I had a sample of the eyelash gel tested independently with a biochemist in Houston and he found ingredients in it that could potentially do what was reported in the company memos."

I took a breath as the words tumbled out in one exhale. I was eager to get back to that slit lamp vendor.

"In addition to data on the Plaintoful eyelash gel, we also found a memo between Ally's ex-boyfriend and the company's VP, Mr. Cooper, discussing the company's malfeasance and giving them both a motive to get rid of

Ally. Therefore, it stands to reason that if they knew that she knew what was going on and was willing to expose it, then the last person to see Ally alive might just be her killer. So, we figured we should have a look into Mr. Cooper's office to see if there was evidence that she had been there at all, and we found it." I stopped speaking and pulled the bag of evidence from Mr. Cooper's room out of my purse.

"What is that?" he asked, staring at the contents of the bag skeptically.

"I found this in Mr. Cooper's wastebasket in his room. It's Ally's eyedrop bottle. I recognized it from all the make-up on it when she showed it to me in my office last week. I even commented on how dirty it was since she carried it in her purse. I can't account for the broken piece of plastic sealant, but the makeup on this tissue matches the eye make-up Ally was wearing. You can have forensics match it, that will prove she was in his room," I said as I handed him the bag of evidence.

"Is that an elastic hair band on the bag? Thi, where did you get that bag?" Lan asked. "That's not another sample from the Vendors' Hall, is it?"

"No, it's from the ice bucket in our hotel room. It's all I had!"

"Girlfriend, you need to be better prepared if you are going to be playing detective," Lan chortled.

"My sentiments as well," Detective Henderson agreed. "In any event, I'm not sure that's enough to accuse him of murder. I'm afraid to ask, but how exactly did you get in his hotel room as you had these two creating a diversion?"

"Let's just say the contact between the locks and the doorjambs don't work that well in this hotel. Also, I found a key bit of evidence on the floor of Mr. Cooper's room. It was lucky that housekeeping hadn't been there yet.

Housekeeping!" I exclaimed. "You need to get up there now and look in his room. On the floor in front of his desk are faint blue scuff marks. The same color as Ally's shoes. If you'll remember what they looked like."

"Whoa. I can't just burst into someone's room based on a questionable search."

"Listen, I am no lawyer, but the marks can be seen on the floor of the room unobstructed and out in the open. I'm just a concerned citizen who happened to notice the faulty lock on the door. Here, I took a picture of it on my phone," I said pulling it up and showing him.

He studied the marks carefully. We all waited anxiously. It was so quiet that when he eventually spoke, we all recoiled at the sound of his voice.

"Okay," he relented letting out a sigh. "I think with all the evidence you've presented; it would be worth at least talking to Mr. Cooper."

"Great. Maybe you can trip him up into confessing!" I exclaimed excitedly.

"Ladies," he uttered taking a breath and trying to maintain his composure. "I'm not promising anything other than a conversation with Mr. Cooper. I appreciate the evidence that you have collected and the interest you have in this case. However, until I get the medical examiner's report on exact cause of death, we can't even fully call it a murder. So, I'll go have a talk with Mr. Cooper."

We all got up and started to follow him.

"Whoa, ladies. Where are you going?" he asked, stopping abruptly.

"We're following you to talk to Mr. Cooper," I said as if it were obvious.

"I think I'd better handle this on my own. If I show up with a mob of angry women, he'll feel defensive and probably lawyer up without saying anything."

"Who are you calling angry?" Adriana snapped.

"And who are you calling a blob?" Lan confronted.

"He said mob Lan, not blob," I explained.

"Oh, never mind then. Carry on," she replied backing down.

"Ladies, I think the situation calls for a cautious and solo inquiry," Detective Henderson informed us.

"I guess you're right," I acquiesced with disappointment.

"How about I let you know how it goes afterwards," he said warming to us.

"That would be great!" I replied clapping my hands with glee for any inclusion. "Until then detective. Good luck."

He went off to Mr. Cooper's room and I headed to the Vendors' Hall and straight to the slit lamp booth where Adriana, Ally and I were at earlier. It was decided that it would probably not be a good idea for Adriana and Lan to return to the Vendors' Hall after their recent activities there. We agreed to meet back at the hotel room later. Luckily, the same company representative was still at the booth when I got there, and he remembered me. I explained the situation and he agreed to let me download the images of Ally's eyelids to my USB drive. When I got back to my hotel room, the others were decompressing with glasses of wine.

"Where did you get that?" I asked.

"We agreed that we earned some libation, so we ordered a bottle to be brought to our room. There's a glass for you," Lan said pointing to the glass on the counter next to the coffee pot.

"I'm too nervous to drink," I replied pacing the floor trying to figure out how Mr. Cooper could have killed Ally with nothing more than a few faint scuff marks on the floor. He certainly seemed strong and cold enough to have pinned her against his desk until she died. However, she surely would have fought back. And Mr. Cooper didn't have a mark on him nor was a hair out of place on that perfectly coiffed head of his. Ally had no marks on her neck to suggest strangulation, but the broken blood vessels on the whites of her eyes did point to asphyxiation. But how do you suffocate someone without squeezing their neck? Finally, what caused that partial circular bruise on her chest?

"Will you stop pacing Dr. Trí? You are making me anxious again and counteracting what the wine is supposed to be doing. Lord knows I need to calm down after that charade we went through in the Vendors' Hall," Adriana declared taking another sip from her glass.

"How *did* you guys pull off such a convincing diversion anyway? You did such a good job, it got everyone to come down and investigate," I commended.

"You know, I just thought about all the money we lost on re-makes from people who think changing an axis two degrees will make a big difference with their eyeglasses, and I let the emotions flow," Adriana replied.

"She was incredible. I just thought about poor Ally sitting there dead on the toilet and it made me angry too. It was easy to feed off Adriana's energy. She was so saucy and loud. I'll stay on her good side from now on," Lan chimed in.

"Lan did a great job of playing a passionate activist. I didn't know she was such a diva," Adriana laughed as she and Lan fist bumped each other.

"Yes, they were great. If I didn't know them, I would have totally thought they were a couple of unhinged tourists or something. I mean look at their outfits. They even looked the part with that orange and gold beaded dress and elbow length, shiny white gloves Lan's wearing. The best part is that headband on your head. Are those plastic eyeballs attached to white lace, ribbons? I mean where can you even get something like that?" Dr. Peregrine laughed.

"I got it out of Thi's suitcase," Lan said candidly and poured herself another glass of wine.

"It's not a headband, it's a fascinator. I call it, "keeping our eyes in the cloud". The white parts of the eyes are acrylic, like what the ocularists use for prosthetic eyes. I'll have you know, the irises are made of dichroic glass to give them an iridescence. They were some of my best works. I thought it was appropriate for this setting," I declared.

"Yes, I see that now. Lovely work." Dr. Peregrine replied uncomfortably. "Well, Adriana's rainbow knitted beanie and scarf just screams activist zealot. All she needed were some matching gloves."

I pulled out the knitted gloves I was wearing to investigate Mr. Cooper's room from my purse and showed them to Dr. Peregrine. They were part of the matching beanie and scarf set I knitted months ago when I was working on Dr. Moore's case.

"Oh. A bit warm for this time of year, aren't they?" Dr. Peregrine asked awkwardly.

"They keep the air conditioning in these hotels high. I get cold," I replied tersely. "And besides, they are a celebration of the color wheel. No political statement intended."

Mercifully my cell phone rang ending the conversation before further feelings were hurt.

303

"Hi Dr. Trí, it's Detective Henderson."

"Yes detective, how did it go? Did he crumble under your inquisition and confess?"

"Not quite. Where are you right now?"

"We're in our hotel next door to the Convention Center. Room 2022. Come on over and give us the news in person."

"I'll be right there," he said and hung up.

"What did he say?" asked Adriana anxiously.

"Not much. He's coming over to tell us."

After a few minutes, which felt like hours, there was a knock on the door. I opened the door to see a somber faced Detective Henderson.

"That is not a face bearing good news," I proclaimed as I stepped out of the way to let him in the room.

"So, he didn't confess?" Lan asked.

"Of course not. He denied knowing how Ms. Gallagher died and was very defensive when I suggested that she had gone to speak to him about problems with his eyelash gel."

"Did you see the scuff marks?" I asked.

"Unfortunately, someone had gotten to them first. The markings were gone."

"He must have cleaned them up after our exchange. Good thing I took pictures," I offered.

"Not sure if those will be admissible in court. I could ask housekeeping if they cleaned them up. However, that's not the worse news I have for you."

"What could be worse?" I asked crestfallen.

"I got word that police officers found the ex-boyfriend, Dr. Brone. A search of his car found Ms. Gallagher's purse in the trunk. He's been taken to the station for questioning. He is our primary suspect."

Chapter 25

H earing that was a gut punch to the system. It felt like being told my diagnosis was wrong and my patient's vision was fading fast.

"Does that mean you're abandoning Mr. Cooper as a suspect?" I asked, the disappointment in my voice was obvious.

"I'm afraid I have no choice. If you give me the paperwork from the company, I could maybe slap him with public health endangerment and criminal conspiracy, but murder? I don't have enough. I'll take the eyedrop bottle and used tissue to forensics to verify they belonged to the victim, but that only proves she was in Cooper's room, not that she left dead. The ex-boyfriend had the victim's purse and was caught heading to the ocean to dispose of it. Forensics also found strands of his hair and his fingerprints on her clothes and person. Those are solid pieces of evidence that he was in physical contact with the victim. You also said she had broken up with him recently. It gives him motive for a crime of passion. We'll know better when we interview him."

"Well can I at least go with you to hear the interview. I'll stay behind the two-way mirror. Pleeeaaase," I begged.

"Okay, but only if you promise not to interfere."

"I absolutely promise. Could I ride with you because I don't have a car here?"

"Fine. Let's go."

"What about us?" Lan asked.

"We have the Genericeye Corporation dinner tonight. Are you still going to come?" Dr. Peregrine chimed in.

"You two, go and enjoy yourselves in the lovely San Diego sunshine," I directed pointing to Adriana and Lan. "I will make it back in time for the dinner. What time is it at, 7:00 p.m.?"

"Yes, but I'll have to be there early to schmooze with industry professionals and the public."

"That you can totally do without me. I'm not good at that anyway, so I'll see you later," I said as I grabbed my purse and headed out the door with Detective Henderson.

As we drove to the police station, we were mostly silent. I was lost in my thoughts about the case. Undoubtedly the ex-boyfriend was involved, but most likely recruited to move the body and get rid of the purse. Why was he driving to the ocean? Why didn't he just dump it in a trash can or leave it with the body?

"You're surprisingly quiet," Detective Henderson said giving me a fleeting sideways glance.

"My husband likes to tell me that it worries him when I'm quiet. At least when I'm talking, he knows what I'm thinking."

"Sounds like a smart guy."

"He is. And very patient and supportive too. Probably why we're still married."

"True enough. Patience and support, the hallmarks of a strong, happy marriage," he said with a tinge of either regret or sarcasm.

"I'm feeling like you are not a fan of marriage. Did you have a bad experience?" I asked curiously.

"I'm not against marriage, but my line of work can be tough on a relationship. Long, unpredictable hours and tough cases can make you less patient and supportive."

"So, I'm guessing you never made it to the alter."

"Almost did, but she decided she would rather have someone she knew for certain would be there for her."

"Sorry to hear that. At least you can take comfort in that it wasn't necessarily a problem with you but more the job," I stated trying to be positive.

"Yeah, there's that," he sneered sarcastically. "Law enforcement can be a tough profession on personal relationships."

"So can optometry."

"What? You docs got it easy. Punch in, look at a few eyeballs, sell some fancy glasses and be home before dinner even gets cold."

"You think so?" I answered feigning enlightenment. "What about the patient that walks in at ten minutes to closing with an angry red eye that they've been self-treating with over-the-counter eyedrops and getting no relief because they have raging, sight-threatening, inflammation? Or the person with a corneal abrasion who went to the ER, was given an eye patch and sent home only to come to the office days later with an infection so bad, they may need a corneal transplant? Then there's the patient with crippling double vision or severe visual distortions that require custom made contact lenses, glasses, surgery, or a combination of treatments. And of course, regardless of the hour of the day, there's the emotional difficulty of telling patients that they have an eye condition that will cause them to permanently lose vision, such as glaucoma, macular degeneration, etc."

"I don't know what most of those words mean," he replied.

"What I'm saying is sometimes we don't get to clock out when the 5 o'clock whistle blows because we need to take care of patients, whether they have sight-threatening conditions or just need a simple pair of glasses, until there's a resolution. And we must do it with professionalism and a smile on our face even if we're dead tired or had a horrible day from being yelled at by the public. Don't you think we take that home with us too?"

"Yeah, I guess that could be a downer."

We were silent again for a few minutes.

"Don't get me wrong," I began, more calmly. "I'm not trying to compare optometry to law enforcement at all. What you all do is tremendously difficult at times. The danger, the uncertainty and sometimes the tedium. I'm just saying there's more to what optometrists, as primary eye care providers, do than just spin a few dials and sell glasses."

"I'm getting that. Sorry to touch a sore spot doc. We're here," he said as he pulled into a reserved parking spot. "Remember, you are just here to observe quietly."

We walked into the police station. It was abuzz with activity. Detective Henderson walked us through the maze of hallways and bustle of people, only briefly pausing along the way to exchange a word or a look with someone. He seemed well respected, which gave me comfort that I was dealing with a competent and professional individual. We worked our way to a questioning room. He directed me into the adjacent observation room.

"Stay here," he said brusquely and went into the other room where the suspect was sitting. Dr. Brone looked exhausted emotionally and physically. His expression was that of a man uncertain of what he should do next.

"I'm Detective Henderson. You have been read your rights. I'm going to ask you a few questions. I understand you were romantically involved with the deceased Ally Gallagher," Detective Henderson asked directly.

"Yes, we were in a relationship," he answered.

"It ended recently?"

"Yes."

"When exactly?"

"Yesterday."

"So, while you were here at the eye meeting?"

"Yes."

"Who broke it off?"

"She did."

"What was the reason?"

"It's personal," he said his face tightening.

"Okay, would you say you were upset that she broke up with you?"

"I wasn't happy about it, but I understood her feelings."

"Did she break up with you over the fact that your company was in the process of covering up questionable side effects of the new eye product?"

"I don't know what you're talking about," he replied shifting nervously in his seat.

"I have in my possession, a memo between you and Mr. Cooper, the vice president of Genericeye Corporation. It discusses questionable side effects with the new eyelash gel product. Mr. Cooper did not want to stop the launch of this product to the public to correct these effects. Have you anything to say about this?"

Dr. Brone looked stunned with this information presented to him.

"I want to talk to a lawyer," he said recovering his composure.

"Okay, you have that right. But let me just tell you that we have enough evidence to charge you with reckless endangerment and criminal conspiracy, which is a felony. You're looking at prison time."

We waited half an hour for Dr. Brone's lawyer to come. As soon as he arrived, the questioning continued. I asked Detective Henderson if I could be in the room during the questioning.

"I don't think that's a good idea. This guy is already tense, what makes you think another person in the room will help?"

"Let's just say, I have a way of getting people to tell me things. If it isn't working, I'll leave. What do you have to lose?"

He gave me a long, thoughtful look and then relented. "Okay, but if things go wrong, you're out of there."

"Understood," I answered dutifully.

We entered the room and sat across from Dr. Brone and his lawyer, who immediately started to look me up and down. A look I was used to from people who were unsure of my abilities based on my physical appearance.

"Who are you?" the lawyer asked.

"I'm Dr. Thi Trí, OD. Who are you?" I responded in a steady tone. I admitted I resented "the look" even though I was used to it. Detective Henderson shot me a look to play nice.

"I am Mr. Ghouls. I am Dr. Brone's lawyer, and you are not law enforcement, so I question your presence here."

"Well Mr. Ghouls, congratulations, you are correct. I am not law enforcement, but I am the person Dr. Brone ran into on his way to find Ally Gallagher before her untimely demise."

"I see," he replied curtly.

"First of all, I just wanted to tell you Dr. Brone that I'm sorry for your loss. Ally was a special person. She was my Genericeye Corporation sales representative you know. Always smiling and positive. She had a great spirit."

"Yes, she did," he replied quietly.

"That day that you were looking for her in the Vendors' Hall. You seemed really agitated. You were certainly anxious to find her quickly. Why was that?"

"I needed to talk to her about something."

"Could you tell us what that was?"

"I'd rather not say," he replied looking at his lawyer, who nodded approvingly.

"I see, maybe personal matters about your relationship. She talked about you to me before the conference."

"She did?" he asked, brightening up.

"Yes, she told me she was excited to have some time off with you, even though it would be working at the conference. She was excited that you would get to be in San Diego together. She thought you might even propose, and she was so happy. I could tell she really cared about you."

These words made his brow unfurrow and his shoulders drop. He was relaxing a bit.

"I can tell you cared about her too. Before you ran into me in the Vendors' Hall, she had run into me first. She told me she was on her way to see Mr. Cooper about something important. She seemed very nervous, scared even. I think she was on her way to tell Mr. Cooper that she knew about the side effects of the eyelash gel and that he shouldn't launch the product yet until there were more safety tests. It's the type of thing she would do because she was such a caring person, right?"

"That was her problem, she cared too much, and she wouldn't listen to me to leave it alone. I was trying to find her to get her to stop. It was too dangerous, and she shouldn't get involved in corporate decisions. That was not our business, but she wouldn't listen."

Mr. Ghouls motioned to Dr. Brone to stop talking. I cleared my throat loudly to bring the attention back to me.

"I know Ally would have wanted to confront Mr. Cooper because it was the right thing to do, but I don't think she would have thought her life was in danger. I mean, why would it be? She was just going to talk to Mr. Cooper, right? He's the vice president of the company, a professional. I met the man. Sharp dresser. Smiles a lot. I mean, what would he have done to her?"

"Mr. Cooper presents himself as a congenial man, but he was dangerous," he said soberly.

"Why is that? I mean, I guess he could have fired her."

"He doesn't like loose ends."

"Do you mean he would not only have fired her, but maybe blackmailed her into silence or something? I mean, I've seen the memo too. I think she knew too much."

"She did know too much."

"And that's what got her killed isn't?"

He stayed quiet but nodded inadvertently.

"Did Mr. Cooper kill her?"

He stayed quiet.

"What sort of man is Mr. Cooper? What lengths do you think he would have taken to keep Ally silent?"

"Don't answer that," his lawyer said.

"I understand that if Genericeye Corporation delayed the launch of Plaintoful eyelash gel and contact lenses over safety concerns, they would have lost millions of dollars. Mr. Cooper strikes me as a man who would take drastic steps to not let that happen. Would you agree with that?"

"Yes."

"Did you have the misfortune to make him unhappy. I know you were part of the lab that worked on the eyelash gel. Did he blame you for the negative results?"

"He was unhappy with the team."

"But you were in charge of the team and the study, right?"

"Yes."

"I'm sure you were working as diligently as you could. I mean the claims for the eyelash gel are quite extraordinary. A real game changer for dry eyes as well as eyelash growth. A health and beauty product in one. That would have been revolutionary."

"Profoundly. We worked very hard on the product."

"But it wasn't ready, was it? Did you try to tell him that?"

"Yes."

"What did he do? Did he try to tell you to falsify the results?"

"Yes."

"Did you?"

"No. I couldn't do it."

"That's commendable of you, but I doubt he would have let it go at that. What *did* he get you to do?"

"He told me to just stay quiet. That he would handle the launch."

"But Ally found out, didn't she?"

"She saw how agitated I was and asked what was wrong. She must have looked through my papers and found the memo.

"Dr. Brone, did you kill her?"

"No. I loved her."

"But you know who did kill her don't you?" Detective Henderson asked.

Dr. Brone stayed silent.

"My client does not need to answer any more of your questions on the grounds that it might incriminate him. He told you he didn't do it and you have no proof that he did," his lawyer said.

"On the contrary, we found the victim's purse in his car. Not to mention his hair on her clothing," Detective Henderson countered.

"That's not much to charge him with," he replied.

"That's enough to hold him until we can get to the bottom of things, and we will get to the bottom of things. Even if we can't prove that he killed Ally Gallagher, we can get him on accessory after the fact since he clearly knows more than he is saying."

"Dr. Brone," I interrupted. "I was the one who found Ally in the restroom at the convention center with my friend. I can say that she was placed there with great care. Her clothes and hair were neat. Even her hands were clasped together instead of left dangling. Her eyes were closed so that she looked as if she was sleeping peacefully. Only someone who cared for her would have placed her in that position, not a cold-blooded killer."

"She deserved as much," he said wiping a tear from his eyes.

"Say nothing more," his lawyer advised.

"Look, I don't know if Mr. Cooper killed her or how she died. I only know that I was told to get rid of the body. But I didn't have the heart to just throw her into the ocean or bury her in the sand."

"So, you put her in the restroom where you knew she would be found," I stated sympathetically.

He nodded and then started to weep silently into his hands.

"I think we're done here," said his lawyer.

"For now," Detective Henderson stated as we rose and left the room. Outside of the interrogation room Detective Henderson let loose some words of disgust and frustration.

"What is it?" I asked.

"Damn lawyers. He was so close to cracking. Without a confession, it's going to be harder to prove that he's our guy since we don't have more solid evidence against him."

"But you heard what he said. He didn't do it. I really feel like it was Mr. Cooper," I remarked.

"All we have is the word of a desperate man. Of course, he's going to deny it and you'll forgive me if I need more than your 'feeling' to arrest Mr. Cooper," he retorted.

"But what about the eyedrop bottle and tissue in Mr. Cooper's trash?"

"It proves she was in the room, not that she was killed there."

I was running out of possible scenarios. I thought back to the clues and information I did have and tried to extrapolate from there.

"There was also a piece of plastic sealant. Did you look at the contents of Ally's purse?" I asked, a hypothesis forming in my mind. I just needed to see if there was data to verify it.

"What about it?" he asked intrigued.

315

"Since Ally threw her artificial tears bottle in the trash, that might mean she opened a new one or was handed one. The piece of plastic is one of those security seals around new bottles. I'll bet there's a new bottle in her purse. She was upset when she bumped into me, she might have even been crying so she would have wanted to put re-wetting drops in her eyes to hide the redness. If there is a brand-new bottle of artificial tears in her purse, we should dust it for fingerprints as well as test its contents."

"I understand dusting for prints, but why test its contents if it's just moisture drops?"

"Just a hunch. Maybe it's just me but why would she throw away a bottle of drops and open a new one when the old one still had some inside?"

"Okay," he acquiesced. "If there is a bottle as you say, I'll do it. Let's go look now."

We went to where the evidence was kept, and Detective Henderson asked for the purse. He turned it upside down and emptied its contents onto a table. There were so many things in the purse. It's true what they say, the bigger the purse, the more stuff we carry in it. There was make-up, a wallet, some brochures, keys, mints, even jewelry. No eyedrop bottle. My heart sank. I was so sure the bottle would be there, and it would be another part of the picture. It didn't make sense that it wasn't there.

"Sorry doc. Nice theory, but I don't see your eyedrop bottle," Detective Henderson stated with subtle disappointment.

"Wait a minute," I asserted suddenly and investigated further into the purse.

"What are you looking for?"

"This," I announced pointing at a zipper for a small pocket inside the purse. I opened it and inside of it was a brand, new bottle of eyedrops. "She probably put it in there to keep it clean since I chastised her for the filthy state her last bottle was in."

Detective Henderson smiled and chuckled to himself.

"Okay, fair is fair. I'll have our forensics team check on it and let you know what we find. I better drop you back at the convention center now so I can get some work done."

Detective Henderson's phone rang, and he answered it. After a few silent moments, he thanked the caller for the information and hung up.

He turned to me and said, "It's official. Ally Gallagher died of asphyxiation."

Chapter 26

I said good-bye to Detective Henderson as he dropped me off at the convention center. I had texted the others that I was heading back there and to meet in our hotel room. I found them there snacking on a room service tray of charcuterie, cheese, crackers, and fruit while sipping sparkling wine.

"Are you guys ordering room service again?" I asked diving in myself.

"Well considering how this trip is a bust for beach trips and fine dining, this is the only luxury we could indulge in," Lan replied wearing an "I love San Diego" tee shirt that she bought at the hotel gift shop.

"So how did it go?" Dr. Peregrine asked eagerly.

"Did Dr. Brone confess?" Adriana added.

"No, he didn't confess to murdering Ally," I replied. "We know he's not the guy anyway, but he did confess to putting her dead body in the restroom."

"If he confessed to putting Ally's body in the restroom, what makes you so sure he couldn't have killed her too?" Dr. Peregrine asked.

"I admit that anyone has the potential to kill someone given extreme circumstances. But I would think those deaths would likely be accidental or in the heat of the moment. If Dr. Brone had killed Ally to try and stop her from talking, I would imagine it would have been in more of a passionate way. For example, he might have grabbed or pushed her causing her to fall and hit her head. Something of that nature. If there was a physical altercation, you would expect there to be more defensive wounds too. Instead, the life was squeezed out of Ally from asphyxiation. That would mean a longer, slower, and more painful death. The killer would be watching to make sure she died, and the way Dr. Brone looked, I can't imagine him doing that. He broke down in tears at the memory of even putting Ally in the restroom. I felt bad for him. I think he really did love her."

"Aw, poor guy," Lan said between chews.

"How can you sympathize with that guy. He is part of a conspiracy to endanger the public and he admitted to helping cover up a murder!" Dr. Peregrine interjected with outrage.

"He said he was following his boss's orders to get rid of Ally's body, and to be fair, he put her in a place to be found," I pointed out.

"So, he admitted that Mr. Cooper killed her then," Dr. Peregrine concluded.

"I knew that guy was guilty!" Lan exclaimed waving her finger in the air and shaking her head.

"No, he said he doesn't know for sure if Mr. Cooper killed her or how she died. He was only told to get rid of the body. But come on, with such a cold, calculating manner and murderous eyes like that? How can it not be Mr. Cooper?"

"But what about Dr. Lassiere? From what I hear, the way he talks to his staff, he could easily commit murder," Adriana offered.

"True, but would he bother to leave her body somewhere to be found?" I countered.

"No, but he could have gotten his efficient manager to take care of it for him," Adriana suggested.

"Intriguing. She does seem like she would do anything for him. Maybe even kill," I wondered aloud.

"So, what do we do now?" Dr. Peregrine asked.

"Let's go through the data and facts of what we know again," I replied. "We know that Ally was in Mr. Cooper's room and that she went to see him shortly before she died. She had no marks on her when we found her except for that circular bruise and some scuffs on her shoes even though the coroner says she died of asphyxiation. Was there anything unusual in the other Genericeye Corporation hotel rooms or that the other sales representative might have said to you Dr. Peregrine?"

"Hmm," she pondered as she thought back to the experience. "The only thing I can think of was there were stacks of samples in their makeshift conference room."

"Makes sense since we're at a conference. They were there to give to eyecare providers."

"But wait, there were also samples of cold and allergy medication," she remembered.

"What was that for?"

"The representative said their company treats more than dry eyes. They also make cold and allergy medicine. They shipped them all together here to save costs. Non-eyecare representatives would pick them up here."

"That's interesting. Anything to save a buck I guess."

"No kidding. He said that they had to reformulate the medication because the earlier version exacerbated respiratory distress in people with predisposed conditions. The company lost millions. It's no wonder Mr. Cooper is so desperate to make it up with the Plaintoful eyelash gel and contact lenses."

"Hmm," I considered. Something about that information tickled my brain and nagged at me. "Was the medication syrup or pills?"

"There were both kinds. Is that significant?"

"Possibly," I answered feeling frustrated.

The answer was at the periphery of my mind's eye. I strained to see it, but it remained a blur.

"Sorry guys. Let's do something else for a while. I have the pictures from the slit lamp salesman in the Vendors' Hall of Ally's eyes. Let's look at it. Maybe it will tell us something," I suggested.

"I have my laptop. I brought it in case I needed to review anything from my studies for Genericeye Corporation's eyelash gel and contact lens launch," Dr. Peregrine said.

We set it up and we all crowded around the screen to look at the images. There was Ally's eye, and there were the lid cells I zoomed into.

"Well, those eyelid cells still look concerning. Looks like her eyes were a bit red too. Seems the eye gel didn't solve her dry eye problems after all," I noted.

"How can you tell that's why her eyes are red?" asked Adriana.

"The blood vessels on the whites of her eyes are engorged, and do you see how the reflection from the white part of her eyes is broken up instead of smooth and even? There is no tear layer. No wonder she needed eye drops.

But she had an open bottle of artificial tears eyedrops. Why would she open a new one?"

"You said her old one was caked with dirt and make-up. Maybe she just wanted to use a new one. Especially in front of her boss," Adriana suggested.

"You could be right," I replied distractedly.

"That's creepy looking," Lan said. "I can't believe you like looking at things like that all day."

"I guess I never thought about it that way. I find the structures of the eyes beautiful. It's an amazing organ really with all types of cells and tissues that make it up. You've got nerves, muscles, blood vessels."

"I get it, I get it," she replied while putting down the piece of cold meat she was holding. She shook with revulsion which threw the sparkling wine in the glass she was holding onto my blouse.

"Ugh, Lan!" I cried. "You spilled wine on me!"

"Sorry Thi!" she exclaimed mortified. "It was an accident."

"I know," I replied. "This is one of my favorite blouses is all. I hope it doesn't stain."

I went into the bathroom and took off my blouse. I laid it on the bathroom countertop, put some water on a washcloth and tried to rub off the wine. I looked up into the mirror in frustration. I could see the lanyard with my convention name tag hanging on the door behind me. As I stared in the mirror, standing half naked, the answer revealed itself to me. Like the final lens drop in a phoropter, the blur disappeared, and everything became clear. All the bits of data came together and were forming one image that jumped out to me. This conclusion, regardless of how unbelievable it was, had to be right. I walked out of the bathroom and into the main room where the others were eating and chatting. I stood there staring at them silently with a serene expression.

"What is it?" Dr. Peregrine asked, noticing my presence.

The others fell silent and looked at me also.

"You figured it out didn't you Dr. Tri?" Adriana asked, recognizing that look on my face.

"Yes, ladies I believe I have. And after confirming a couple of things with Detective Henderson, we're going to catch ourselves a killer tonight."

"Tonight?" asked Dr. Peregrine. "But the Genericeye Corporation dinner is tonight."

"Exactly. All the players will be there tonight. It's time for the end game."

Chapter 27

T

hat evening, Dr. Peregrine and I dressed up in our best attire and headed to the dining hall where the Genericeye Corporation Plaintoful product launch dinner was being held. Lan and Adriana had to content themselves with drinks at the hotel bar. As we found our seats, Dr. Peregrine was visibly nervous. Her hands trembled and she was constantly fidgeting with her purse.

"Would you relax?" I told her.

"That's easy for you to say. You don't have to contend with the fall out after you potentially cause the downfall of a major eye health corporation. Are you sure you know what you're doing?"

"Pretty sure. I mean I never accused anyone of murder to their face, in public before. But it can't be much worse than dealing with belligerent patients."

"I mean, are you sure you have the proof and everything?"

I looked around the room. There at the front tables, close to the podium, was Dr. Lassiere looking dapper in a suit and tie complete with his circular tie pin. Seated alongside him was his stern manager, Ms. Paine. She wore a dark blue dress and her ever-present gold company brooch. At the podium area where the speakers would be talking, was Mr. Cooper impeccably dressed as usual. He was wearing a navy blue, three-piece, suit and crisp black, buttoned-down shirt. His tie was tucked into his vest and his cufflinks sparkled under the fluorescent lighting.

"Yes, yes I do," I assured her.

The room filled up quickly with several hundred attendees. The house lights flickered to indicate everyone should be seated and that the first speaker of the night was about to begin. I looked across the room to the doors but the only people there were the wait staff. I looked down at my watch. He should have been here by now, but hopefully will be here soon. The first speaker was a public relations person for Genericeye Corporation who put up slides and videos describing how wonderful the Genericeye Corporation was and how they were continuing to innovate and be the industry leaders. It was a shame that their company was being led by an unscrupulous person, otherwise they sounded like a solid company. After about twenty minutes of self-congratulations, the speaker introduced Mr. Cooper. He stood at the podium and adjusted the microphone to his stature. He looked out at the crowd with all the confidence of a man with nothing but success. By the end of his speech, I looked over at the main door and saw Detective Henderson enter. At the side doors two other uniformed policemen entered and stood guard.

"And in conclusion, our new eyelash gel and accompanying contact lenses will be a game changer in the eye industry. And we at Genericeye Corporation are the leaders that are bringing it to you. Are there any questions?" he asked as the room erupted into applause.

"Yes, I have a question," I projected as loudly as I could while standing up.

Mr. Cooper looked over to me and the smile disappeared from his face as he recognized me. "Yes, Dr.?" he asked pretending to forget my name.

"It's Dr. Trí, sir. We met earlier today when I was asking you about one of your Genericeye Corporation's employees, the late Ms. Ally Gallagher who most tragically died here at the convention," I announced looking all around the room to make sure everyone could hear me. Dr. Lassiere turned in his chair at the mention of Ally's name. He and Ms. Paine stared at me intently.

"Yes, I remember you," he said glibly. "You were snooping around our hotel rooms trying to play detective or something I imagine. You know optometrists are only supposed to look into eye problems, not solve deaths. I believe that's out of your purview."

Dr. Lassiere and Ms. Paine snorted and smirked at the jab while others were surprised and uncomfortable with the statement.

"True, investigating homicides is beyond our scope of practice, but you see Ally Gallagher was a good person. She always treated me right even though I am but a humble optometrist in a small private practice," I responded shooting a cutting look at Dr. Lassiere and Ms. Paine. "So, I took it upon myself to help solve her murder, because in fact she was murdered most cruelly by you."

A collective gasp and shock swept the room at my words. Even Dr. Lassiere and Ms. Paine were surprised as all eyes were glued on Mr. Cooper and me.

"What is this nonsense? You had better stop and consider what you are saying before you find yourself in legal peril, doctor," he insisted coldly having dropped the façade of congeniality by now.

"I have nothing to fear when the truth is on my side Mr. Cooper. I doubt you can say the same. You see Ally Gallagher found out about the dangerous side effects of the Plaintoful eyelash gel which can potentially cause eyelid cells to turn cancerous."

Another collective gasp swept the room.

"She had already started to suspect the eyelash gel was dangerous after using it herself for several months and noticing a change to her eyelids. She gave me a sample of it, knowing I would probably have it checked out. And I did have it analyzed by an independent biochemist at the University of Houston, who confirmed its synthetic growth compounds are potentially carcinogenic. But it was when she arrived at this convention that she found the memo between you and your head researcher on the Plaintoful product, Dr. Brone. It confirmed a cover up by Genericeye Corporation. You instructed Dr. Brone, who wanted to delay the product launch to ensure its safety, to stay quiet while you proceeded with the launch in order to save millions of dollars on press that had already been spent. Despite Dr. Brone trying to convince Ally to stay quiet, she scheduled a meeting with you in your hotel room to confront you with the cover up. I have the memo along with pictures of her eyelid and data from your labs to confirm all of this."

"Okay I can say that maybe there are a few wrinkles in the Plaintoful eyelash gel formulation that still need ironing out, but we are already working on it. Let me assure you all that the product is safe and ready to use," he smiled at the crowd. "As far as the murder accusation, what proof do you have of that? As I understand it, she didn't have a mark on her to indicate foul play. I mean, how would I have even done it? So maybe you should write up all your ridiculous theories in a book and end it with how you trashed your insignificant optometric career by accusing the vice president of a multi-billion dollar company of murder without any evidence."

"Wow is your tie tied too tightly because that was incredibly rude. You should loosen that tie anyway, because I've read that wearing a tie too tightly can cause your eye pressure to go up. You wouldn't want glaucoma, would you?" I jabbered awkwardly and took a sip of water to steady my nerves. My anxiety was at crisis level with so many eyes upon me.

"Get on with it," Detective Henderson blurted out trying to disguise it as a cough.

"Right, anyway. Let's talk theory. You knew that Ally was meeting you to talk about Plaintoful's side effects because you had a heads-up from Dr. Brone. So, when she arrived you had already formulated a plan to silence her. We found a brand, new bottle of artificial tears in her purse as well as a piece of plastic sealant in your trash this afternoon with your fingerprints on both."

"I admit I offered her a new bottle of artificial tears when she came to see me. She was upset, her eyes were red, and she was going to put drops in her eyes from a very dirty bottle, so I offered her a clean one. If anything, I'd say I saved her from an eye infection."

There were a few chuckles from the crowd.

"Why that would be admirable of you, if it were just artificial tears, but in fact it was medication from one of your company's cold and allergy products. The very same that in high enough concentration is contraindicated in people susceptible to respiratory illness because it was shown to severely aggravate the condition. With your biochemistry background, it would have been easy for you to crush up some of your company's medication and compound it into innocent looking eyedrops. When Ally used it, it was only a matter of time before it killed her."

"Now I know you've lost your mind. How could I possibly put cold and allergy medicine into a tiny little bottle of artificial tears?" he laughed.

"By squeezing out all the former solution from the bottle and then using the empty bottle to suck up the new dangerous concoction the way you would suck up solution with an eye dropper. It wouldn't be too difficult to do, am I right doctors?" I asked addressing the crowd of optometrists in the room.

Some of them nodded their heads in agreement while others murmured approval of my speech so far.

"Anyhow. When she showed up, you offered her the new bottle of artificial tears because you knew she had dry eyes from the form she had to fill out to be part of the clinical trials for the Plaintoful eyelash gel. She threw her old bottle away and took your bottle, used it, and then put it away in her purse."

"Even if this happened, and I'm not saying it did, she was a perfectly healthy person. Our medication was changed to a milder form. It wouldn't have been enough to kill her, but maybe cause her some discomfort as she was trying to cause me and the company. Besides, my hotel suite is right next door to a common room. None of my employees heard a peep," he replied smugly.

"True, perhaps that delivery system would have limited systemic absorption. However, what you didn't know was that just a few minutes earlier, Ms. Paine of Southeast Texas Lasik Center, had given her allergy medication. The two together would have produced a tremendous effect. Even so, had she been a healthy individual without any predisposed health conditions, perhaps the medications themselves wouldn't have killed her. But when she left me in the Vendors' Hall on her way to see you, she was already very nervous causing her heart rate to go up and affecting her breathing. This is because she didn't just have 'dry eyes', but she had Sjogren's Syndrome, which is an autoimmune disorder that causes dry eyes, dry mouth, and in some cases, can affect the lungs.

Therefore, by using your eye drop concoction, enough of the medicine drained through her tear ducts and into her blood stream, adding to the medication that was already in her system. Her respiratory system then went into dangerous levels of distress. While she was struggling to breathe, you pinned her against the desk in your hotel room. She was in such a frantic and weakened state that she was unable to fight back or even catch her breath enough to scream. You held her arms down with your left hand and with your right arm pressed against her chest. Then you leaned with the weight of your body against her to prevent her from inhaling air and essentially caused her to suffocate. The scuff marks on her beautiful blue shoes and on the floor below the desk in your room indicate she was struggling to get out from under you. However, in her weakened state, she couldn't. It wouldn't have taken much effort to stop her breathing. You wouldn't even have had to muss up your perfectly coiffed hair."

Mr. Cooper started to clap his hands in a mocking way. An insidious smile covered his face.

"That is a most creative way to kill someone. Except, you don't have proof to show that I even touched her.

From what I hear, Dr. Brone is in custody. He was her jilted lover after all."

"We have the tainted bottle of artificial tears with Ally and your fingerprints on it. And as far as the proof that you held her down until she was dead, you're right. I don't have the proof on me, but you do. You see her body wasn't completely without a mark when she died. She had a crescent shaped bruise on her chest that was made peri-mortem. Since she didn't have that mark on her when I saw her an hour earlier in the Vendors' Hall, I knew it must have been made by the killer. I initially thought it was perhaps part of a circle from a pendant, a button, tie pin or even a brooch. But Ally didn't wear any such type of pendant and no one else had any of those items that correctly fit the shape and size of the bruise. Because the curve faced right and the opening faced left, I didn't make the connection that it was in fact not an incomplete circle, but the letter "c" backwards. And this letter "c" looks just like the one on your shiny, gold, monogrammed cufflinks."

The collective gasp in the room quickly went from horror to anger. Cries of "murderer!" were echoing in the room. Mr. Cooper looked down at his cufflinks and his expression turned from cool mockery to panic as he turned to flee.

However, as he attempted to run, Dr. Lassiere tackled him to the ground. Then he raised his fist and punched Mr. Cooper in the face saying, "That's for Ms. Gallagher you scumbag!"

Detective Henderson and his men rushed over to separate the men and handcuff Mr. Cooper before Dr. Lassiere could do anymore damage.

Dr. Peregrine was looking incredibly relieved as she slumped back in her chair and fanned herself with her napkin. I continued standing for some reason. Then I locked eyes with Dr. Lassiere who gave me a partial smile and a nod that wordlessly conveyed, "respect". Someone started clapping in a slow and rhythmic manner. This induced others to start clapping as well until the whole room erupted with applause, whistles, and the occasional shouts of "way to go doc!". I must admit, it felt good to have solved the case and to have brought justice for Ally. I kept standing and soaking in the accolades because frankly, after all the bad events that had happened to me and my office last week, I deserved it. I may not be the most successful optometrist, or the greatest detective, but I'm sure I'm the best optometric detective around. Under 5'6" anyway. I smiled and gave an awkward bow to my peers. Thankfully the wait staff started bringing out our dinner. Dr. Peregrine and I enjoyed our well-earned meal, complete with extra desserts offered to us by some of our tablemates.

We left the dining hall in a state of food coma and went to the bar to find Lan and Adriana. They were sitting at the bar counter with drinks in their hands. They were laughing and chatting with a couple of good-looking men when we approached.

"Ahem, how's your husband doing Lan?" I asked out loud, which made the men scurry away.

"Dr. Trí! What did you do that for? I'm not married!" protested Adriana.

"Sorry Adriana. I'm in food coma, wasn't thinking," I replied sheepishly.

"How did the reveal go? Did you catch the murdering bastard?" Lan asked loudly. She had clearly been drinking for some time.

"I did indeed," I said proudly. "I even got a positive acknowledgement from grumpy Dr. Lassiere."

"No way," laughed Adriana. "That's awesome. Congratulations. You earned it."

"She was brilliant," Dr. Peregrine added. "I sensed there was a moment when you were losing your nerve, but you pulled it out in the end."

"What? Me, nervous? Never," I lied. "I'm just glad Mr. Cooper was still wearing the same cufflinks that he had on when he murdered poor Ally."

"I'm sad to have missed it," Lan sulked.

"I saw a few people with cameras out. I think you might find it on social media somewhere," I laughed.

"Probably. This is a crazy world we live in. People can't even confront murderers in private anymore. So, what happens now?" Lan asked.

"Shouldn't you be telling us?" I replied sarcastically. "Isn't your husband a cop?"

"Yes, but we don't talk about what happens after he catches the perp. We're usually in the bedroom by then," she grinned.

"Ooh, girl," laughed Adriana as she clinked her wine glass to Lan's.

"Detective Henderson will match the size and shape of Mr. Cooper's cufflinks to Ally's bruise as well as have forensics swab for Ally's DNA. A positive result, along with Dr. Brone's testimony should be enough for a conviction."

"And *we* fly home tomorrow for a vacation from our vacation," Lan exclaimed as she drank down the rest of her glass of wine.

"Not us," Adriana said sadly.

"We start work at our new jobs at Dr. Moore's office," I added woefully. "Back to our day jobs."

Chapter 28

B

ecause several attendees from the convention were on our flight home, we were inundated with chatter about what Mr. Cooper's arrest would mean for Genericeye Corporation. The most popular speculation was that their stocks would take a nosedive in the immediate aftermath, but then they would probably re-brand or maybe even be absorbed by a competitor. That seems to be the way with these companies.

I couldn't wait to get home and tell Fred about all that had happened. Evidently, he had already heard some of it from the news. Someone had indeed filmed my exchange with Mr. Cooper on their smart phone and posted it on social media, which was picked up by the news stations.

"How does it feel to be a hero?" Fred asked as I walked in the door.

"I'm not going to lie, it feels pretty good," I gushed happily. "Like when I give a child their first pair of glasses and they see what they've been missing in their blurry haze, except cranked up a thousand times better."

"Well, you were always my hero *and* a hero to those children getting their first pair of glasses," he said giving me a big hug. "I imagine you'll be famous at work tomorrow. Maybe you could negotiate a few days off, just to recover a bit. We could drive out to that little bed and breakfast outside of Austin that you like. I watched that video of you online, so I knew you were nervous."

"Maybe so. I thought I hid it relatively well. Anyway, there's no way Dr. Moore is going to give me time off any time soon."

The next morning, I drove to Dr. Moore's office with my white coat washed and starch pressed. It was a rarity for me since I usually just washed, dried, and fluffed my clinic jacket. A stiff white jacket was so formal. However, I wanted to make a good impression on my first day. When I drove into the parking lot, I noticed a huge crowd of people around the front of the office. Some had microphones and cameras.

"Uh oh, reporters," I surmised.

I drove to the back side of the office and parked out of view. I hurried to the back door of the clinic with my sunglasses on and my head held down and knocked on the door. No one came to the door, so I knocked again and then I noticed the clinic's security camera overhead. I took off my sunglasses and looked up at the camera and waved my hands. A few moments later, a staff member opened the door, hurried me in and quickly locked the door again. We were in the break room and there were the sounds of chaos out in the front of the office. Adriana was already there and pouring herself a cup of coffee. I was glad to see a familiar face.

"Good morning, Adriana. What is going on out there?" I asked.

"Good morning, Dr. Trí. Yeah, it's chaos. Somehow the reporters found out that you work here. They were here waiting an hour before we opened according to the other occupants of the mall."

"Ugh, our neighbors must not be too happy that they're taking up parking spots and causing traffic."

"They'll get over it. It's free publicity for them. It's Dr. Moore who you should be worried about. The phone has been ringing off the hook for people wanting to schedule an appointment with you. Even the patients who already had appointments with other doctors are wanting to switch to see you. Some of the younger staff are freaking out and asking to go home."

"And to think I was nervous about remembering where the bathroom was. First days. You've got to love 'em," I grumbled.

Dr. Moore came bursting into the break room. He was red in the face and flustered.

"Go home," he said as he came over to me.

"But I just got here," I protested.

"Nothing is going to get done today so long as you are here. These reporters are refusing to leave until you come out and talk to them. Why don't you take a few days off until this madness dies down," he commanded.

"Really?" I asked incredulously.

"Really," he replied emphatically.

"I helped Dr. Trí catch the bad guy, maybe I should take a few days off too," Adriana offered.

"Not a chance. You're supposed to be the optical manager, go out there and manage this situation!" he ordered.

Adriana quietly took her cup of coffee with her and left the break room. I shot her a sympathetic look.

"Look at it this way, it's free publicity for the clinic," I offered.

He pursed his lips, flared his nostrils, and pointed towards the door. I left and hurried home. Fred was delighted to hear that I had a few days off and we quickly made our escape before the reporters showed up at our house. Luckily, we were on good terms with our neighbors, and they chased off anyone who came around that didn't belong.

After a few days, the excitement about the hometown hero died down and I found myself deeply ensconced in the exhausting pace of seeing many patients every day. If my old clinic had seen as many patients in a month as we did here in a week, Adriana and I would have decided to rebuild our little clinic. But I had to admit, being free of administrative and financial responsibilities gave me more time for patient care. And if some patients wanted to complain about insurance and fees, I could just send them off to the billing department to take care of it there.

Another bonus in the first few weeks was that my notoriety afforded me adoration and respect from my patients and the staff. However, as the months went on, the novelty and luster wore off and I soon found myself feeling burned out as the abuse returned from unruly patients. The staff went back to sniggering at me behind my back and catering to the other doctors that had more influence in the clinic. My patients were often attended to last, which put them in bad moods by the time I got to them. I even had a few patients refuse to see me based on my race and gender. The staff tried to hide this from me, but the loud manner in which the patients spoke echoed throughout the clinic.

Adriana was doing well. Her overall knowledge of the optical, clinic equipment, insurance and other facets of optometric business made her an essential person and popular with staff who were less experienced. It also raised the ire of the more senior staff. Office politics reared its ugly head, but Adriana ever the diplomat, assuaged their concerns for job security. We were sad that we didn't get to see each other as often in the day and talk as we used to.

One day, as I finished an exam and was ready to take my lunch break, Adriana found me to let me know I had a phone call.

"Is it Fred?" I asked, not knowing who else would call me at work.

"Nope. It is a blast from the past. The mother of one of our old patients," she smiled wryly.

"You're scaring me," I said feeling my mouth going dry.

"It's Mrs. Stableson. The mother of that young man who didn't want to play football anymore based on your recommendation."

"And the father who excoriated me severely, and unfairly I might add."

"That's the one."

"What does she want?"

"Sorry Dr. Trí, but she didn't want to tell me. She just wanted to talk to you, but she didn't sound angry. More apologetic really. You can use the phone in the lab. The break room is a cesspool of gossip."

"Okay, thanks."

I went into the lab. It smelled of burning plastic, but at least the lab tech and opticians had taken a break for lunch, so it was quiet. I steadied myself, picked up the phone receiver and pressed the blinking light that went to line 2.

"Hello, this is Dr. Trí. How can I help you?"

"Hi Dr. Trí. This is Mrs. Stableson, Mike Stableson's mother. Do you remember me?" the voice on the other line said hesitantly.

"Yes, of course I do. How are you doing?"

"Honestly, not great, but trying to get better."

"Sorry to hear that. Is there anything I can do?"

"I should have listened to you and maybe things would have been different," she said passionately, her voice breaking as if she were going to cry.

"What's happened?" I asked very concerned at this point.

"My son continued to play football since his father insisted. He wanted him to get a scholarship to a big sports school and turn professional someday. But a few months ago, during a game, he got sacked very hard. He wasn't getting up, so they took him to the hospital. He ended up having a cerebral hemorrhage. They had to put him in an induced coma to treat it."

"Oh, my goodness! I'm so sorry," I exclaimed in shock.

"Thank you. Anyway, he came out of it a week ago and so they transferred him to TIRR in the medical center for his recovery. They say that he's lost some of his vision from the injury too, so he's working with a Low Vision specialist and an occupational therapist to adapt to his new condition. I mentioned your name and the optometrist knew you."

"Oh yes, I worked there as one of my clinic rotations during my Low Vision residency. The Low Vision specialty within optometry is a small community, so we're aware of each other."

"She had nothing but good things to say about you, which made me think to call you. I wanted you to know what happened to my son. He was always so fond of you. I tried to call your old office, but the number has been disconnected. I looked you up online and saw that you had moved to this office."

"Yes, unfortunately my old office burned down in an unfortunate accident. Adriana, my office manager, and I decided not to rebuild so I took a job here instead."

"I'm sorry to hear that. We liked your little office, despite the disagreements over football."

"Thank you. I miss it from time to time but can't dwell on the past. It's best to focus on the future and not to worry about what you can't control."

"This is true. But you're happy in your new job?"

"Happy enough. It's very busy here. Much busier than at my old office so I guess I'm a little worn out. I'm more of a worker bee here. It's an adjustment when you're used to being in charge if you know what I mean."

"Yes, I think I do. Can I ask you a question?"

"Sure."

"Do you think you would be happier working for a non-profit? I imagine the pace would be slower."

"I never really thought about it. I guess if the right opportunity came up. Why do you ask? Do you know of a job?" I asked flippantly.

"As a matter of fact, I do. The Low Vision optometrist at TIRR says there's a position open at the Diminished Vision Center near Montrose. We were just chatting, and she said they tried to recruit her, but she was happy where she was. You should give them a call. I am a donor and my mother sat on their board years ago. I would be happy to give you a recommendation."

"Wow, that's very kind of you. Thank you. I'll think it over and let you know."

"This number that I called on is my cell number. Call me if you change your mind."

"I will do that. Thank you, Mrs. Stableson. And please say hello to your son. I know they'll take good care of him at TIRR," I assured her as I quickly wrote down her phone number from the caller ID and slipped it into my clinic jacket pocket.

"Good luck to you Dr. Trí. Goodbye," she said and hung up.

I hung up the phone just as Adriana popped her head into the room.

"You all right in here? You've been in here so long you don't have much time left for lunch."

"It's the weirdest thing," I said ruminating on what just transpired.

"What happened? I hope she didn't call just to chew you out again."

"No, she called to let me know that her son kept playing football and ended up in the hospital with a cerebral hemorrhage. He's even lost some of his vision."

"Oh my god!" she exclaimed.

"He's past the crisis point now and is recovering at TIRR thank goodness. The interesting twist is that she wants to do me a good turn now. She told me about a Low Vision specialist position at the nonprofit, Diminished Vision Center. She said she would give me a recommendation for it if I wanted the job."

"Do you want the job? It's been a while since you did any Low Vision, but I know you had always wanted to do some at our office."

"True. We never started it at our office because of the extended time that it requires with patients, and we just didn't see enough of those types of patients. Honestly, I think I'm burning out here. The pace is too quick, and the patient load is too full. Also, the office politics is demoralizing. I feel like the low woman on the totem pole. I hate to say it, but I'm struggling."

"I hear you Dr. Trí. I overheard the staff saying they think you're too slow. But I think the other doctors are too fast frankly. I know I'd want more than ten minutes with my doctor."

"Right?" I replied, happy to have a sympathetic ear. "But I wouldn't want to leave you here by yourself in this den of vipers."

"Don't worry about me. For me, it's just work. I don't take it personally. I know it bothers you, as it should. Times have changed. People used to have more respect for their doctors. I know if I put in as many years of school as you all have, I wouldn't like people yelling and harassing me every day. So, if you're unhappy here, go somewhere better for you. I think those blind people, ..."

"Visually impaired," I corrected her.

"Excuse me, visually impaired people would benefit greatly from your care. You like to take the time with patients to really help them. As much as it drove me crazy, I was glad for it. So maybe this job is exactly what you need."

"Well, I'll have to think about it," I said hesitantly.

We could hear a male patient being led to the pre-work up room. He was talking to the staff.

"My doctor's a woman, eh? I hope she's attractive because I like to get my money's worth in my exam."

Adriana and I exchanged similar glances of disgust. She pointed to the phone. I picked up the receiver and dialed Mrs. Stableson's number.

"Hello, Mrs. Stableson. This is Dr. Trí. I'll take you up on that offer for a recommendation. I'd like to apply for that Low Vision job at Diminished Vision Center."

What's next for Dr. Thi Trí, O.D.?

Join Dr. Thi Trí, O.D. on her next cases when she leaves the cutthroat, money-driven, corporate world for the clandestine operations of non-profits. When a seemingly healthy Low Vision patient falls dead in her waiting room and a prominent surgeon is killed in his office, Dr. Trí will need her special insight to investigate two deaths in, *A Non-Profitable Murder.*

About the Author

Dorothy Mai spent her formative years in Los Angeles, California when her family arrived from Vietnam at the end of the Vietnam and American War. After obtaining a B.S. in Molecular Biology at the University of California, Los Angeles, she moved to Houston, TX to attend optometry school at the University of Houston, College of Optometry. Like her fictional character Dr. Thi Trí, O.D., Dorothy Mai is an optometrist who works in the Greater Houston area. She is residency trained in Low Vision and Rehabilitation. During her optometric career, she has worked in a multitude of optometric clinical settings. These settings include: an ophthalmology group, private and corporate optometry practices, non-profit organizations and at the University of Houston, College of Optometry. While at the College of Optometry, she participated in and presented research at several optometry meetings and has published research in several peer reviewed journals.